Traditional Chinese Medicine in the United States

Traditional Chinese Medicine in the United States

In Search of Spiritual Meaning and Ultimate Health

Emily S. Wu

LEXINGTON BOOKS
Lanham • Boulder • New York • Toronto • Plymouth, UK

Published by Lexington Books
A wholly owned subsidiary of The Rowman & Littlefield Publishing Group, Inc.
4501 Forbes Boulevard, Suite 200, Lanham, Maryland 20706
www.rowman.com

10 Thornbury Road, Plymouth PL6 7PP, United Kingdom

Copyright © 2013 by Lexington Books

All rights reserved. No part of this book may be reproduced in any form or by any electronic or mechanical means, including information storage and retrieval systems, without written permission from the publisher, except by a reviewer who may quote passages in a review.

British Library Cataloguing in Publication Information Available

Library of Congress Cataloging-in-Publication Data
Wu, Emily S., 1978–
Traditional Chinese medicine in the United States : in search of spiritual meaning and ultimate health / Emily S. Wu.
p. ; cm.
Includes bibliographical references and index.
ISBN 978-0-7391-7366-4 (cloth : alk. paper) — ISBN 978-0-7391-7367-1 (electronic)
I. Title.
[DNLM: 1. Medicine, Chinese Traditional—United States. WB 55.C4]
R733
610—dc23
2013012284

ISBN 978-1-4985-1510-8 (pbk : alk. paper)

∞™ The paper used in this publication meets the minimum requirements of American National Standard for Information Sciences Permanence of Paper for Printed Library Materials, ANSI/NISO Z39.48-1992.

Printed in the United States of America

Contents

Preface		1
Introduction		5
1	Geography, Demographics, and General Trends	15
2	Evolution of TCM in the Bay Area	29
3	Knowledge Transmission and Identity Formation of an "Alternative" Medicine	45
4	TCM Healers in the Chinese Community	75
5	TCM as Complementary Medicine	89
6	TCM as an Alternative Medicine	103
7	Creating a Space for Psychic Healing	117
8	Going to the Culturally Authentic	133
9	Healing, Environment, and Lifestyle Changes	147
10	The Happenings in an Acupuncture Clinic	163
11	The Embodied Spirituality of *Qi*	171
12	Ideal Body and Concept of Health	189
13	Concluding Analysis	203
Appendix		217
Bibliography		229
Index		233
About the Author		237

Preface

This book tries to answer a seemingly simple question: "What is traditional Chinese medicine?"

It is a simple question that could be investigated from many vantage points. This book does not represent the vantage points that seek scientific and medical explanations or justifications for traditional Chinese medicine (TCM); nor does this book, based much on fieldwork in the San Francisco Bay Area and on survey in California, represent TCM on a global scale. Instead, this book focuses on the social aspects of TCM as the medical theories and practices are translated and interpreted by TCM practitioners who are situated in the American context.

In the ensuing chapters, I hope to demonstrate the fluidity of a medical ideological system with a rich history of methodological development and internal theoretical conflicts, which continues to transform in our postmodern world where people and ideas transcend geographic, ethnic, and linguistic limitations. The transnational, transcultural reality of TCM is evident in my study of the TCM practitioners in the Bay Area. It is not a medical system that exists only "out there," over in a far-away corner of the world, nor is it merely the remnant of a glorious ancient civilization. The unique historical trajectories and cultural dynamics of the American society are precious nutrients for the localization of TCM, while the constant traffic of travelers and immigrants fosters the globalizing tendency of TCM. The practitioners I interviewed for this project therefore represent an incredible range of clinical applications, personal styles, theoretical rationalizations, and business models.

What really unifies all these practitioners is not their practices, but the goal of these practices. The shared goal is to strive for health, not just health in terms of the lack of illness, but the ultimate health of achieving perfect balance in every aspect of the being of a person—physically, mentally, spiritually, and energetically.

Therefore, the simple answer to the seemingly simple question is this: on the most basic level, TCM is where people try to somehow calibrate into perfect balance. The rest of the book consists of how that answer makes sense in the context of the modern world with decreasing distances and diminishing boundaries between cultures.

PERSONAL BEGINNING AND ACKNOWLEDGMENTS

For many decades in the twentieth century, my grandfather was the only Western biomedical doctor in my hometown in rural central Taiwan. Since he was one of the very few highly educated people among the mostly illiterate farming population in our town, there were few he could have an intellectual conversation with. When he was in his eighties, my grandfather was a grumpy old man who rarely smiled. With eyeglasses as thick as the bottoms of soda bottles, he spent most of his days reading medical journals in Japanese, watching Chinese opera on television, and cursing in German (nobody else in the household knew any German). He believed that his training in medicine and science gave him a far superior perspective on the world than everyone around him. This was especially true, at least to him (evident from the constant bickering between him and my grandmother), when it came to the argument of who got to choose the channel to watch on TV.

My grandfather notoriously had only one friend on the street where we lived. Across the street from us was a traditional Chinese herb shop. The herbal doctor who owned the shop, also in his eighties, was the only person on the entire street my grandfather would talk to outside our own family. I was often sent over to the medicine shop to walk him home for dinner.

The herb shop was dimly lit and filled with the smell of chopped, powdered, and sometimes boiled herbs. In the glass display case were tied batches of dried seahorses, several pairs of deer antlers, and tin cans of ginseng imported from Korea. On the giant cabinet behind the counter were rows of tin cans previously used for milk powder, now labeled with names of herbs and minerals. The surface of the wooden counter was darkened and beaten, and across the counter sat the two old men, similarly weathered but conversing vibrantly as if age had forgotten them. They would drink right at the counter, and those were the only times I ever saw my usually stern and severe grandfather laugh. Later he would walk home with a package of herbs, a gift from his dear friend to make his favorite tonic soup.

Back at my house, my father also practiced as the only Western doctor in town, in the clinic my grandfather had established. Much more down-to-earth and approachable than his father, my father, with the assistance of my also-medically-trained mother, often made home visits to patients who were unable to come to the clinic. In the 1980s, when Taiwan was fast developing into a more industrial nation, our little farming town's population consisted mostly of elderly people and the grandchildren under their care. As a responsible family physician, my father dedicated the following twenty-five years of his life to educating his patients about how to take better care of their health. Over the years, his patients also taught him much about folk healing practices that came largely out of necessity, as they tried to solve their health problems while also struggling with poverty and old age.

The elderly farmers sometimes had remedies that were passed down through their families, or told to them by their neighbors and friends. Sometimes when they made a trip to town to visit my father's clinic, they also hopped across the street afterward to get some Chinese herbs. First upset by his patients' medical infidelity, my father gradually learned to monitor their health while taking their herb consumption into consideration. He never understood the full scheme of traditional Chinese medicine, nor did he intend to actively incorporate it into his own practice. However, his conversations with patients were sometimes speckled with terminologies that did not belong to Western medicine. Patients often could not differentiate between Western and Chinese medical models, and he became used to descriptions such as "my chest feels stuffy, like there is stagnated central *qi*" (*himkam zaza, diongki buisoon*胸脯實實,中氣不順; in hokkien dialect) or "I told him not to eat too much hot food; now his nose is bleeding because there is too much heat in his body."

Sometimes, when my non-Chinese practitioner informants learned that I spent my childhood in rural Taiwan (or other times, just because of the mere fact that I speak English with a very slight Chinese accent), they asked me if the way they practiced was anything like "how it's done authentically." The assumption seems to be based in the Orientalist fantasy of that isolated paradise where true Chinese medicine fully constitutes the daily healthcare of everyone. The assumption is not entirely false; culturally and linguistically, I did have much more exposure to some of the ideas and terminology that permeated the daily speech and behaviors in the life of rural Taiwan. Vaguely and almost intuitively, I understood the physical experiences of conditions such as excess heat (getting unusually thirsty and hot, and the sensation seems to come from the inside) or deficiency of *qi* (tired, lethargic, and unwilling to move). We often had local medicinal herbs in our chicken soup for dinner.

On the other hand, even in rural Taiwan, the medical scene in my upbringing was dominated by Western biomedicine. Being part of the East did not exempt my small hometown from the dominance of biomedicine, and I also happened to live in the only household in town that provided the biomedical services! The popular medical-assistance-seeking protocol, whether it was my own family or our neighbors and friends, had been that biomedicine took care of the urgent and quickly identifiable illnesses and injuries, and Chinese medicine would serve to complement, most commonly by means of herbal formulae or dietary rules. In short, even in my rural life in Taiwan, Chinese medicine was the supplemental, the alternative, the backup, much like the way many Americans utilize TCM in their own healthcare today.

In the late 1980s, half of my household washed ashore in North America on a wave of immigration. While my father stayed behind to continue practicing family medicine in rural Taiwan, my mother accompanied my younger brother and me to be educated in British Columbia, then California. We became jet-setting transnationals, with homes on both sides of the Pacific Ocean, social networks on both continents, and keen awareness of global politics. It was in our diasporic context that my mother decided that she wanted to go back to school and study Chinese medicine. She was forty-three years old and spoke only enough English to buy groceries. There was a weekend program she found in San Francisco that was taught in Chinese, and the professors were all from Mainland China. My mother had been a registered nurse in Taiwan, and she was exempt from a number of elementary science and fundamental biomedicine courses.

This actually became my first real and extensive exposure to Chinese medicine. My mother and her classmates spent countless hours studying at our house; somewhat conveniently, I became the human guinea pig when they needed to practice acupuncture point locations and needling techniques. When my mother eventually acquired the state license and established her own small practice, like many Chinese families that start businesses with the cheap or free labor of their relatives, I became the part-time clinic manager.

And from there my new journey began, not as a daughter of medical practitioners or a clinic manager, but as an academic, a listener and observer, and a storyteller.

This project started with research for my doctoral dissertation, which would not be possible without the generous support and selfless sharing of my TCM practitioner informants. I am also infinitely grateful for the intellectual training and emotional encouragement from my dissertation committee—Judith Berling, Edmond Yee, and Robert Weller—who have continued to support me as mentors, discussion partners, and friends. In order to transform the dissertation into a publishable book, I reached out to Keping Wu, Ofelia Villero, Natalie Quli, and Edmond Yee (again) for theoretical and editorial advice; they suffered through my much-less-than-perfect manuscript and gave preciously honest suggestions. Sophia Park has also been a source of intellectual, emotional, and spiritual guidance in the long process. Catherine Burns has supported me with friendship, *qigong*, and knowledge in medicine, as well as providing ideas and the actual props for the book cover photos. At Lexington Books, Justin Race graciously offered me the opportunity to publish my work, and Sabah Ghulamali has been nothing but patient and insightful in guiding me through the publication process. And finally, I thank my family members, blood-related or otherwise, here physically or in afterlife, for their loving, caring, massaging, talking, and feeding that fueled my body, heart, mind, and spirit.

Introduction

Traditional Chinese medicine originated from the traditional medical system in the Chinese civilization, with influences from the Daoist and Chinese folk traditions in bodily cultivation and longevity techniques. In the past few decades, TCM has become one of the leading alternative medical systems in the United States. In the year 2001 alone, 2.1 million adults in the United States used acupuncture treatments.[1] California was one of the first states to regulate TCM practitioners, who were, and still are, licensed as acupuncturists. In 1972, the state of California started regulating the practice of acupuncture under the supervision of biomedical physicians; by 1978, acupuncturists in California were already established as primary care providers (who require neither supervision nor referral by biomedical physicians).[2] Approximately half of all licensed acupuncturists in the United States currently practice in California.[3] By May 2009, a total of 13,110 acupuncture licenses had been issued in California, more than double the count of 6,300 licenses in 2000.[4] Approximately one-fifth of all licensed acupuncturists in California are currently practicing in the San Francisco Bay Area.[5]

Categorized as complementary and alternative to the dominant biomedicine and as a type of holistic medicine, TCM has enjoyed the status of a popular yet marginalized medical system. Its relative lack of Western scientific evidence for its efficacy seems to be compensated for by its label as a holistic medicine, which takes the spiritual dimension into the consideration of human health. On the other hand, the sophistication of TCM as a historically comprehensive medical system may have contributed to the increasing use of acupuncture while other complementary and alternative medicine (CAM) providers are seeing a decline of visits over the past decade.[6] A July 2009 report from the U.S. Department of Health and Human Services indicates that between 1997 and 2007, visits to acupuncture treatment increased threefold, culminating at 17.6 million visits for the year 2007 alone.[7] Although acupuncture is covered by many health insurance providers, the out-of-pocket cost for 2007 acupuncture usage in the United States was estimated to be at $827 million.[8] In turn, the acupuncture practices in the San Francisco Bay Area alone account for at least $174 million of out-of-pocket costs annually,[9] with healthcare insurance payments contributing significantly more to that figure. To give a sense of the scale of the acupuncture economy in the Bay Area, its estimated annual out-of-pocket cost alone is more than four times the entire annual enacted budget for Healthcare Services (including public healthcare programs such as Medicare and Medi-Cal) in California for the fiscal year of 2009–2010.[10]

The high density of licensed acupuncturists in the San Francisco Bay Area, combined with the continually growing demand for acupuncture treatments, unsurprisingly produced an extremely competitive market for the practitioners of TCM. According to a small-scale California-wide survey I conducted in 2006, 44 percent of the practitioners were Chinese ethnics, and another 41 percent self-identified as of Caucasian/European descent.[11] Caucasian American practitioners must compete with practitioners trained in China, who are deemed culturally authentic and theoretically authoritative. On the other hand, the Chinese immigrant practitioners also often find themselves struggling to adjust to the culturally, linguistically, and ideologically embedded demands and needs of mainstream American patients. The competition is also framed by the unique population composition in the Bay Area—besides being an ethnically diverse population, here also exists one of the most established and politically influential Chinese ethnic communities in the United States. Strong human, economic, and political connections both locally and overseas constantly position the members of this Chinese ethnic community amidst transnational and multinational communications and exchanges. The rich diversity among the members of this Chinese ethnic community also contributes to coexisting and often competing narratives. Most importantly, the depth and breadth of Chinese ethnic influences in the Bay Area necessitates power dynamics that go beyond the mere linear hierarchy typically present in Caucasian-dominant mainstream America.[12]

WAYS TO CONSIDER "TRADITIONAL CHINESE MEDICINE"

Many of the TCM practitioners I talked to were quick to point out the dubious nature of the term "Traditional Chinese Medicine." Along with some scholars who study practitioners of Chinese medicine in Mainland China and in the United States,[13] my informants reminded me that the conception of "traditional" Chinese medicine is a recent and highly politicized project, where "traditional" was controlled and reconstructed by the Communist government. It is, caution some Caucasian American practitioners, a system sterilized of the potentially spiritual language and concepts that were previously abundant in the classical Chinese medical literature, and the remaining materials became merely survival strategies implemented by barefoot doctors during the Cultural Revolution.[14]

In the context of People's Republic of China (PRC), TCM is a state-regulated medicine. With "superstitious" elements eliminated, clinical efficacy supported by scientific research, and epistemology explained with biomedical categories and criteria, there exists a PRC vision of modernized indigenous medicine that is equivalent to and capable of being integrated with biomedicine, and is able to provide modalities that are often drastically less costly than Western biomedical treatments.[15]

In the context of China as a civilization, traditional Chinese medicine is a culturally embedded medical system that includes a wide range of theoretical paradigms and practical strategies for healthcare for all dimensions of human existence. Physical, emotional, interpersonal, astrological, mathematical, spiritual, and ritual techniques were and are creatively utilized. The plurality of this medical system is unified by some general ideological assumptions that are products of a long history of dialogues, debates, cross-referencing, and borrowing between intellectual schools (literary, political, and religious teachings included). In short, it is a system that is internally diverse and constantly evolving.[16] Concepts such as *qi* 氣 and theories such as *yinyang* 陰陽 and the five elements (*wuxing* 五行) are commonly used to explain and understand the mechanisms on various levels of human existence.[17]

There are also conceptual implications in how medical practitioners are labeled and categorized in the Chinese language. The character *zhong* 中 means "center" or "middle," which is usually the shortened form for China (*zhongguo* 中國, or the Middle Country) or Chinese (*zhongguoren* 中國人; person of the Middle Country). *Yi* 醫 could mean medicine, practitioner of medicine, healing, or the healer. The two characters combined, *zhongyi* 中醫 can possibly be understood as: 1) Chinese medicine; 2) medicine(s) of China; 3) a doctor or practitioner of Chinese medicine, including acupuncturists, herbalists, and practitioners of other modalities; and less commonly, 4) a doctor who is ethnically Chinese, regardless of what type of medicine. Frequently, *zhongyishi* 中醫師 is used to identify a doctor of Chinese medicine, and to differentiate the practitioner from the biomedical paradigm.

The term *xiyi* 西醫, where *xi* 西 means West or Western, also stands for "Western medicine" and "practitioner of Western medicine." Interestingly, while *zhongyishi* is used to identify a doctor in Chinese medicine, the term *xiyishi* 西醫師 is never used. Instead, when people use the generic term for doctor, *yishi* 醫師 or *yisheng* 醫生, they generally mean a doctor who practices Western medicine. In other words, a doctor of Western medicine is the "standard" doctor, and a doctor of Chinese medicine needs to be indicated as such. By implication, Western medicine is considered the standard medicine, and Chinese medicine is identified by differentiating from and contrasting to the standard.

The "traditional" part of "Traditional Chinese Medicine" and "traditional Chinese medicine" is only marked when the term *chuantong* 傳統 (traditional) is used in conjunction, as in *chuantong zhongyi* 傳統中醫. In everyday Chinese speech, it is not common to have to identify *zhongyi* as *chuantong zhongyi*, unless it is contrasted against a more modern form of *zhongyi*, which usually implies that the Chinese medicine is integrated with Western medicine, or *zhongxiyi jiehe* 中西醫結合, which literally translates to "Joint Chinese and Western medicine." There is no modern Chinese medicine, or *xiandai zhongyi* 現代中醫, that is without the Chinese-Western integration.

In the context of the United States, within the predominantly biomedical framework, traditional Chinese medicine, as mentioned before, is a complementary and alternative medicine (CAM). Furthermore, the "traditional" and "indigenous" labels also contrast with the assumed "modernism" of biomedicine. Not only is traditional Chinese medicine indigenized in the American context, but the profession has also reconfigured itself to serve functions that venture into the realms of the psychological, the religious, and, as I argue in this book, the spiritual as well.[18] Categorized under the umbrella of CAM, practitioners of TCM in America, especially but not exclusively those who are not Chinese ethnics, often incorporate the central beliefs and values of the general CAM into their practices and ideology—Holism, Vitalism, spiritual usage of secular language, understanding of health as a state of optimal conditions rather than only the absence of symptoms, and the teamwork relationship between healer and patient.[19] In turn, key concepts in TCM, such as *jing* 精, *qi* 氣, *shen* 神, and the relationships and interactions between *yin* and *yang* and between the five elements, are interpreted through the lenses of the above-mentioned CAM ideologies. Clinical strategies and treatment techniques are similarly explained and justified. More broadly, through interactions and exchanges with other medical systems in its proximity, traditional Chinese medicine also "assimilates and transforms concepts, models, and practices from other medical and non-medical traditions, just as it constitutes itself a resource of techniques and ideas for appropriation by other cultural formations."[20] The complex power dynamics between biomedicine, CAM, and TCM in the American context will be discussed in more detail in later chapters.

In the context of the Chinese American community, traditional Chinese medicine is part of the Chinese cultural heritage that goes beyond clinic visits. The medicine then includes rules and cultural conceptions for daily diets and behaviors, cultivation practices, and other strategies to maintain health.

In the attempt to answer the question of "What is TCM?" in the following chapters, I will use the terms traditional Chinese medicine, Chinese medicine, and TCM interchangeably to include all the interpretations of the term listed above. The interpretations are rarely mutually exclusive, so I will use the terms universally and specify individual incidences as necessary. Whereas some scholars and practitioners argue that TCM stands for the standardized Chinese medicine coming out of the People's Republic of China, I will specify that subcategory as PRC-TCM.

RESEARCH METHODOLOGY

The fieldwork research that supplies the bulk of the data used in this book was done in the San Francisco Bay Area. From April 2008 to December 2011, I conducted formal, in-depth interviews with thirty-five TCM practitioners. Narratives collected from these interviews became the primary source of data in this book. It is unfortunate that my Human Subject Protocol forbids that I identify my informants by their real names, because they really should be individually recognized for their knowledge, their wisdom, and the courage to speak their minds.

In terms of participant observations, I observed in classes and clinics in two acupuncture schools for about two months, and observed in a private clinic for about three months, both toward the end of 2008. I also had observation sessions in several other private clinics, and had informal conversations with practitioners, instructors, and students whom I encountered, some during my intensive fieldwork in 2008–2009, others as early as 2006 and 2007 in social occasions and professional conferences. Some practitioners who contributed perspectives to this research were friends and acquaintances from my fifteen years of residence in the Bay Area, with whom I have conversations and discussions on an occasional but ongoing basis. This supplemental group of informants represents at least fifty more voices in the TCM community in the Bay Area.

I also attended some public events in the trade, such as conferences, school open-houses, and public lectures. These events were rich resources in understanding the most trendy topics, ongoing discussions, and shared concerns of the TCM practitioners.

Again, all of my informants are identified by pseudonyms. Rather than referring to them by full names, I identify them by names that are consistent with the way that the individuals prefer to be addressed in real life. For instance, most of the non-Chinese practitioners refer to themselves by their given names, while Chinese ethnic practitioners sometimes prefer to be addressed as Doctor, Daifu, or Yishi (both "Daifu" and "Yishi" mean doctor in Chinese), even if by California law they are not considered doctors unless they have obtained a doctorate in Oriental Medicine.

Finally, all quotes from the classical Chinese texts cited in this book are my own translations from Chinese originals unless otherwise noted.

OUTLINE OF THE BOOK

This book starts with a larger picture of TCM in the American context — where the TCM practitioners in this study are located, who they are as a group, how the TCM profession has evolved in its short history in the Bay Area, and how the practitioners are trained. To provide the context within which the TCM discussed in this book arises from, chapter 1 outlines the general geographic and demographic landscape of the San Francisco Bay Area, as well as the survey results that describe the statistical information of TCM practitioners in California and in the Bay Area. Temporally, to present a sense of how TCM transformed historically in California, chapter 2 portrays the life stories and narratives of four acupuncturists who represent different generations of TCM practitioners who served the Bay Area community. Based on observations and interviews at local TCM schools and clinics, chapter 3 describes how TCM practitioners are trained by various official, supplemental, and personal transmissions of medical knowledge and clinical skills. The issue of the formation of the professional image and identity of the practitioners will also be discussed.

Chapters 4 through 10 provide personal narratives and close observations of TCM practitioners in the Bay Area. Practitioners share stories about their journeys finding and building their individual preferences in how they practice TCM. Their previous professions, other trainings, and experiences figure greatly into how they conceptualize TCM as a medical system and how they each translate and interpret medical knowledge into actual clinical practices. Chapter 4 showcases the voices of those practitioners who specialize in TCM modalities that are popular in the Chinese ethnic community—acupuncture, herbology, manual treatments, and ritual healing. These practitioners are so heavily in demand among Chinese diasporans that they mostly do not need to venture beyond the cultural and linguistic confines of the local Chinese ethnic community, even when they have non-Chinese patients coming to them. Chapters 5 through 8 present groups of TCM practitioners who orient themselves between biomedicine, TCM, and other sources of healing powers and knowledge. The first two groups practice TCM as complementary (chapter 5) and alternative (chapter 6) to biomedicine, which is consistent with how the National Institute of Health categorizes TCM.[21] The practitioners in chapter 7 are blessed with strong intuitions and psychic powers and use TCM modalities in conjunction to create a legitimate space in which they also utilize their otherwise-controversial healing powers. In chapter 8, the already-skilled practitioners explore classical Chinese medical texts to find culturally authentic interpretations to healing, especially in what truly holistic healing might entail. After each orientation of practitioners, there is a recap section to summarize key features in the narratives of each practitioner, and of the practitioners as a group that shares the orientation.

Chapter 9 evolves around an interesting finding—that among practitioners in my study, there is a discourse of environmental awareness and an emphasis on creating a certain type of clinical environment. Practitioners not only reference popular American conceptions of environmental protection; some also incorporate traditional Chinese understandings of how humans relate and interact with nature, particularly from classical medical understandings of the correspondence between the human body and the cosmos.

To supplement the findings in chapters 2 through 7, as well as to provide separation between informant-oriented narratives and the more textual-oriented discussion in chapters 8 and 9, chapter 10 gives a more in-depth and comprehensive impression of the work of one practitioner and the daily operations of her clinic in the Bay Area.

Chapters 11 and 12 build upon the narratives and observations in earlier chapters with an exploration of the conception of the human body and health in classical Chinese medical and philosophical texts. As I will demonstrate in these two chapters, "spiritual" is difficult for the Chinese ethnics to talk about because there is a lack of directly parallel vocabulary in the Chinese language. Significantly, then, the concept of *qi* 氣, the cosmically shared energetic material, is an important entry point into talking about the spiritual dimension of human existence. This *qi*-oriented understanding of the body is not limited to the Chinese ethnic practitioners—it is shared by TCM practitioners cross-culturally. The implications of this paradigm is that health is not just lack of symptoms of injuries and disease, or even just stability in the bodily system; ultimate health in TCM is a state of perfect balance and self-sustainability that one can only strive for, a state that is in fact impossible to reach and maintain.

Finally, chapter 13 concludes the book with analysis of how TCM practitioners in the Bay Area have transformed both the theorizations and applications of TCM as they actively participate in the movements of globalization. As transnationals who have resources in multiple cultural and knowledge systems, the practitioners make TCM a medicine that works for their patients, in their own unique ways.

NOTES

1. See National Center for Complementary and Alternative Medicines (NCCAM, part of the National Institute of Health) website: http://nccam.nih.gov/health/acupuncture/#ususe (accessed August 28, 2009).

2. See State of California Department of Consumer Affairs Acupuncture Board website: http://www.acupuncture.ca.gov/about_us/history.shtml (accessed August 28, 2009).

3. See Hans A. Baer, *Toward an Integrative Medicine: Merging Alternative Therapies with Biomedicine* (Walnut Creek, CA: AltaMira Press, 2004), 49.

4. The licensee count for 2000 can be found in the University of California, San Francisco, commissioned vocational report on Acupuncture, 2004. I arrived at the May 2009 license count by going directly to the license verification engine, accessible for the general public, on the State of California Acupuncture Board website, http://www2.dca.ca.gov/pls/wllpub/wllqryna$lcev2.startup?p_qte_code=AC&p_qte_pgm_code=6500. More about statistical information of licensed acupuncturists in the Bay Area can be found in the next chapter.

5. See chapter 1 for more information.

6. Although several Asian indigenous medical systems (Korean, Japanese, and Vietnamese) use acupuncture as one of the treatment modalities, the licensing exams for acupuncture in the United States are based exclusively on TCM materials. Therefore, although there are acupuncture schools in the United States that teach non-TCM acupuncture, most schools now either focus exclusively on TCM or make other medical systems supplemental to the predominantly TCM curricula.

7. See Richard L. Nahin, et al., *Cost of Complementary and Alternative Medicine (Cam) and Frequency of Visits to Cam Practitioners: United States, 2007* (U.S. Department of Health and Human Services, Centers for Disease Control and Prevention, and National Center for Health Statistics, 2009), 4. According to this report, visits for acupuncture treatments went from 27.2 visits per 1,000 adults in 1997 to 79.2 visits per 1,000 adults in 2007.

8. Nahin, et al., 6.

9. This figure is derived from the statistics in Nahin's CDC report with consideration that California acupuncturists account for about half of all licensed acupuncturists in the United States, and one fifth of California licensed acupuncturists are in the Bay Area. In the same report, it indicates that the average out-of-pocket cost per visit for acupuncture is $39.59. This is most likely an underestimation of the real market share value in the Bay Area.

10. See California State budget website, webpage on enacted budget for Healthcare Services 2009–2010: http://www.ebudget.ca.gov/Enacted/StateAgencyBudgets/4000/4260/department.html (accessed October 25, 2009). The enacted 2009–2010 fiscal year budget for California Healthcare is $40,138,962.

11. See appendix, table 2.

12. See chapter 1 for in-depth discussion on cultural dynamics and assimilation models.

13. See Linda L. Barnes, "American Acupuncture and Efficacy: Meanings and Their Points of Insertion," *Medical Anthropology Quarterly* 19, no. 3 (2005): 239–66; Mei Zhan, "Does It Take a Miracle? Negotiating Knowledges, Identities, and Communities of Traditional Chinese Medicine," *Cultural Anthropology* 16, no. 4 (2001): 453–80; Volker Scheid, *Chinese Medicine in Contemporary China: Plurality and Synthesis* (Durham; London: Duke University Press, 2002); Elizabeth Hsu, *The Transmission of Chinese Medicine* (Cambridge; NYC; Melbourn: Cambridge Uinversity Press, 1999).

14. Personal communications, 2008.

15. See Hsu, *The Transmittion of Chinese Medicine*; Scheid, *Chinese Medicine in Contemporary China: Plurality and Synthesis*.

16. See Nathan Sivin, *Traditional Medicine in Contemporary China* (Ann Arbor: Center for Chinese Studies, University of Michigan, 1987); Philip S. Cho, "Ritual and the Occult in Chinese Medicine and Religious Healing: The Development of Zhuyou Exorcism," dissertation (University of Pennsylvania, 2005); Paul U. Unschuld, *Medicine in China: A History of Ideas* (Berkeley; Los Angeles; London: University of California Press, 1985).

17. *Yinyang* and the Five Elements (Metal, Wood, Water, Fire, and Earth) are fundamental theories in Chinese philosophy that go back as far as the Han dynasty (206 BCE–220 CE). They are used to first describe patterns and cycles observed in nature, but the resulting rules extend to all realms of human existence—the functions of the human body, interactions between people, landscaping and geomancy, politics, etc. For a brief explanation of *yinyang* and Five Elements theories, see Livia Kohn, *Daoism and Chinese Culture* (Cambridge, MA: Three Pine Press, 2001), 44–47; for medical application of the Five Elements theory, see Ted. J. Kaptchuk, *The Web That Has No Weaver: Understanding Chinese Medicine* (New York: McGraw-Hill, 2000), 437–52.

18. Linda L. Barnes, "The Psychologizing of Chinese Healing Practices in the United States," *Culture, Medicine, and Psychiatry* 22 (1998): 413–43.

19. See Michael S. Goldstein, "The Emerging Socioeconomic and Political Support for Alternative Medicine in the United States," *Annals of the American Academy of Political and Social Science: Global Perspectives on Complemetary and Alternative Medicine*

583 (2002): 44–63; Bonnie B. O'Connor, *Healing Traditions: Alternative Medicine and the Health Professions* (Philadelphia: University of Pennsylvania Press, 1995); Peter A. Clark, "The Ethics of Alternative Medicine," *Journal of Public Health Policy* 21, no. 4 (2000): 447–70; J. A. English-Lueck, *Health in the New Age: A Study in California Holistic Practices* (Albuquerque: University of New Mexico Press, 1990). Holism here is defined as the belief that the whole is greater than the sum of its parts, with emphasis on individual differences and complexity of factors causing illness, and a deliberate break from mind-body dualism. Vitalism consists of beliefs that there is a life force that suffuses the human body, which is health and healing promoting when it is sufficient and balanced, and illness inducing if blocked or unbalanced.

20. Volker Scheid, "Remodeling the Arsenal of Chinese Medicine: Shared Pasts, Alternative Futures," *Annals of the American Academy of Political and Social Science: Global Perspectives on Complementary and Alternative Medicine* 583 (2002): 137. Also see Hans A. Baer et al., "The Holistic Health Movement in the San Francisco Bay Area: Some Preliminary Observations," *Social Science and Medicine* 47, no. 10 (1998): 1495–1501; Barnes, "The Psychologizing of Chinese Healing Practices in the United States"; Elizabeth Hsu, "The Reception of Western Medicine into China: Examples from Yunnan," in *Science and Empires*, ed. Patrick Petitjean, Catherine Jami, and Anne Marie Moulin (Amsterdam: Kluwer Academic Publishing, 1991); Scheid, *Chinese Medicine in Contemporary China: Plurality and Synthesis*; Claire M. Cassidy, "Chinese Medicine Users in the United States Part I: Utilization, Satisfaction, Medical Plurality," *Journal of Alternative and Complementary Medicine* 4, no. 1 (1998): 17–27.

21. See webpage of National Center for Complementary and Alternative Medicine (NCCAM), part of National Institute of Health: http://nccam.nih.gov/health/whatis-cam/chinesemed.htm.

ONE
Geography, Demographics, and General Trends

This chapter is intended to provide a sketch of the backdrop of this study—the geographic and demographic context, the history of Asian communities in the area, the power dynamic between the Chinese ethnic community and the mainstream American society, and some quantitative survey results collected from TCM practitioners from across California. The TCM practitioners who share their stories and perspectives in the next few chapters are all active participants in this specific context of historical, social, political, and cultural atmosphere.

GEOGRAPHIC AND DEMOGRAPHIC CONTEXT: THE SAN FRANCISCO BAY AREA

As one of the most popular travel destinations in the world, San Francisco is famed for many things—the bright red Golden Gate Bridge, the hilly streets with cable cars, the air of liberalism and hippie creativity, the historical association with the gold rush, and the rich array of ethnic heritages. While tourists usually only visit parts of the downtown area of San Francisco, like all major metropolitan cities in the United States, the San Francisco Bay Area extends far beyond just the city of San Francisco itself. Along the strip around the bay, the downtowns of Oakland, San Francisco, and San Jose serve as main economic and political cores for their respective surrounding regions. While the history of intellectual leadership and avant-garde activism is closely linked to the cities of San Francisco and Berkeley, the high concentration of technology companies in the Silicon Valley (also known as the South Bay) also contributes to the uniqueness of the Bay Area culture.

The U.S. Census Bureau has the San Francisco Bay Area (hereafter referred to as the Bay Area) covering a much larger area than local conception, with no less than nine surrounding counties, and at times counting eleven counties that reach far into central and inland California. Realistically, this Greater Bay Area does share the same metropolitan cores; residents of the peripheral counties often make long commutes to work in the core regions. Therefore, in this study, especially in terms of statistical descriptions, I include the ten counties that surround the inner bay of the Bay Area: Alameda, Contra Costa, Marin, Napa, San Francisco, San Mateo, Santa Clara, Santa Cruz, Solano, and Sonoma (see Appendix, Figure 1). Most of my informants, especially those in whose clinics I observed, are located in the core regions.

As one of the financial centers of the world and a major cosmopolitan area, San Francisco is among top rankers in terms of GDP and real estate values. Even when the real estate values hit rock bottom across the nation as a result of the 2008 financial crisis, some neighborhoods in the core regions of the Bay Area were still holding their values up in the multimillions. Real estate agents lament a "slower market" compared to the crazed sales a few years back. "In the good old days, buyers were so competitive that they routinely add on top of the asking price," an agent who specializes in a luxury neighborhood recounts. "Now they just wait until the price gets a little lower." That "little lower" was still consistently about three times higher than the national average price of single homes at the end of 2008, according to the National Association of Realtors.[1]

The ethnic diversity of the Bay Area today is both the result of the long history of local ethnic enclaves and the cause of a continued influx of migrants who are attracted by the diversity. As California was first colonized by the Spaniards in the 1500s and formally part of Mexico, the Hispanic and Latino presence in the Bay Area began far before the region was even considered "American." Italian, Irish, and Chinese enclaves have existed in the Bay Area for as far back as the late 1840s, when the gold rush attracted immigrant laborers from overseas. In the 1880s, the first significant wave of Japanese migrants came to the Bay Area mostly by way of Hawaii. Korean workers also came by way of Hawaii in the 1900s. Filipino farm laborers were found in the area as early as the 1920s. The Vietnam War brought the Bay Area not only Vietnamese immigrants, but also refugees from Vietnam's neighboring Cambodia and Laos. In the late 1940s, the removal of the Japanese community from the city to concentration camps created a sudden demand for laborers, and brought in 40,000 African-descent workers, mostly migrating from other parts of the country. And of course, people of European descent (besides Italian and Irish), the "invisible" ethnics, have also migrated in from other parts of the United States, from Canada, and from overseas, since the days of the gold rush.

Despite racial discrimination that has at times legally denied the basic rights of some groups—for example, the Chinese Exclusion Act (1882–1943) and Japanese internment during WWII—ethnic-specific enclaves have continued to thrive and exist in the Bay Area to this day. It is important to note that the boundaries between ethnic enclaves may seem rigid on census records, but on the personal level, people of different ethnicities have always worked alongside one another. Friendships and marriages across ethnic lines also create families, whether in blood or in heart, that further blur divides between enclaves. Finally, the rise of the suburbs brought middle- and upper-middle-class people from all ethnicities alike to the new developments, efficiently extending and diluting the ethnic enclaves.

Besides ethnic diversity, the Bay Area is also diverse in many other respects. As a known politically leftist area compared to the rest of the state and the country (especially the metropolitan cores, which can be described as having the range of liberal-progressive-radical), the multitude of lifestyles, ideologies, and identities present in the Bay Area are not only tolerated but also often celebrated. For instance, San Francisco is known for having one of the largest homosexual and queer communities in North America. Major religious traditions, new religious groups, and folk religious practices are widely represented in the area as well. A religious master once told me that all religious groups should have a center in the Bay Area, because that is where every religious group is represented, at least on the West Coast.

THE CHINESE ETHNICS IN THE BAY AREA

The Chinese have been continuously present in California for more than 160 years. After the first wave of laborers for the gold rush in 1848, more Chinese workers came to help build the transcontinental railroad in 1865. For the most part, early Chinese immigrants in California were laborers, fishermen, and merchants from Southeast China. While some children of these pioneer families became professionals and intellectuals, a number of students from Mainland China stayed behind in California after the establishment of the People's Republic of China (PRC) in 1949. Another significant influx of Chinese students who sought graduate and professional education in California did not happen until the 1960s. These students from Taiwan (many of whose families had migrated from Mainland China to Taiwan during or after WWII) were in a different socioeconomic category. Although many worked low-paying labor jobs in Chinese restaurants while they were in school, their educational credentials and fluent English quickly opened doors to upward social mobility.

The Vietnam War brought refugees from across the Indo-China region, and among the refugees were Chinese ethnics. This group is rarely mentioned in the history of Chinese Americans in general. While the Chinese communities in Southeast Asia are known for their close adherence to and observation of the Chinese traditional etiquette, it is not clear how they self-identify ethnically in response to the U.S. Census. Many in this category are from families that have been transnational in Southeast Asia for many generations, and were often born and raised outside of China proper. Furthermore, the ethnic diversity in Indo-China means that many of the families may be ethnic hybrids with Malays, East Indians, and Europeans. They are often multilingual to start with, and are able to participate in different dialect groups both within and outside of the Chinese community in the Bay Area. As a result, they are often merged into the head counts of these dialect groups.

The economic boom in the 1980s brought a wave of entrepreneurial immigrants from Taiwan and Hong Kong. The fear of Hong Kong's return to People's Republic of China's rule in 1997 prompted many Hong Kongers to migrate to North America, with Vancouver and San Francisco (two cities with large Cantonese-speaking populations already established) as favorite destinations. This wave of immigrants was distinctly different from the earlier Chinese immigrants in that they were already upper-middle class before they came, and that economic advantage also gained them political influence rather quickly. The children of these immigrants, both those born overseas and those born in California, were provided with excellent education and financial resources.

Postwar chaos, the Cultural Revolution spanning through the decade between 1966 and 1976, and the closed-door policy of Communist rule kept immigrants from Mainland China very low for nearly three decades. The open door policy of 1978 steadily reintroduced immigrants from the People's Republic of China into the Bay Area, starting mostly from the southern provinces. As transportation technology advanced and global travel became common, immigrants from all over China crossed the Pacific Ocean to find their new homes here. According to the 2000 U.S. Census, 7.4 percent of the total Bay Area population self-identify as Chinese ethnics.[2] The city of San Francisco has the largest Chinese population in the Bay Area, with 20.7 percent of its total residents being Chinese ethnics in 2000.[3]

It is important to recognize that, with the Bay Area's rich diversity, the Chinese ethnics in the Bay Area do not consist only of new immigrants or those who are "fresh off of the boat." Pioneer immigrants made their homes in the Bay Area, and so did the many who followed over the 160-year history of Chinese American presence here. Generations of the oldest families were born and raised here, constantly joined by newcomers, whether legal or illegal, in poverty or in wealth. Chinese Americans from other parts of the country and transnationals from other Chinese ethnic communities around the globe have also continually migrated into the Bay Area. With the complexity of its current structure and the variance in its members, the Chinese population in the Bay Area is an ever-growing mosaic with vibrant colors, and makes tremendous contributions to the general culture of the Bay Area.

As the Chinese ethnic population started to include members from a wide range of home regions and backgrounds, more recent scholarship in Chinese American studies has begun to recognize the importance of class identity in understanding the characteristics of Chinese American communities.[4] Incidentally, class distinctions among Chinese ethnics manifest in the different types of Chinatowns in the Bay Area. Dialect groups also create their own niches, and the sense of community and mutual support often stem from the shared dialects. On the other hand, it is ultimately the socioeconomic position of the customers that decides what merchandise is sold in the stores, or vice versa, where a store that carries goods of certain quality and price range can attract a particular demographic of customers.

The Chinatown located in downtown San Francisco is one of the oldest and most prominent in the country. Dating back to the 1850s (destroyed in the 1906 earthquake and rebuilt thereafter), this Chinatown, along with the old Manhattan Chinatown in New York City, have become the iconic symbols of the history of Chinese immigrant communities in the United States.

The significance of this Chinatown is not only in its impressive history, but also that it has been the prototype of Chinese communities in North America up until recent decades. Furthermore, it remains the home, physically and emotionally, of some Chinese American organizations that have branched out to other parts of the nation. Chinese American scholar Joe Chung Fong observes:

> the social structure of the Chinese community emerged from San Francisco Chinatown. Later, other Chinatowns from the surrounding cities like Sacramento and Stockton modeled themselves after San Francisco's social institutions. As pioneer Chinese immigrants migrated to the continental United States' interior, they patterned small and large Chinese communities' social structure after San Francisco Chinatown. It is no accident that even today the majority of the district and family associations' headquarters are located in San Francisco. Even the progressive American-born Chinese civil rights organization, the Chinese American Citizen League, started in 1895 in San Francisco. Now this organization has many branches in the United States but the Grand Lodge continues to be in San Francisco's Chinatown.[5]

Although Chinatowns used to be the equivalent of a Chinese ethnic enclave, it is important to note that the vast majority of the Chinese ethnics in the Bay Area currently reside in the suburbs all over the Bay Area. Peter Kwong, whose 1996 study focused on the Chinatown in New York City, categorizes contemporary Chinese in America into two socioeconomic groups:

Uptown Chinese, who are better educated and more financially capable than American average, and live away from Chinese-concentrated areas, and **Downtown Chinese**, who are still doing low-wage manual and service jobs, and live either within or in close proximity to the traditional Chinatowns.[6]

Kwong estimates the latter group to make up about 30 percent of the Chinese ethnic population in his New York City sample.[7]

In the Bay Area, the boom of technology-related industries in the Silicon Valley in the 1990s attracted a large inflow of highly educated Chinese ethnic professionals from both abroad and from other parts of the United States. Steady growth of this particular community over the last decade first significantly shifted the proportions between the "Uptown" and the "Downtown" (although Silicon Valley is south of San Francisco), but the demands for services by the "Uptown" professionals attracted yet another inflow of the "Downtown" labor and service providers. Clusters of plaza-style Chinese shops blossomed not only in the South Bay, but also in the East Bay and the Peninsula, around suburbs where Chinese ethnic professionals reside in high concentrations. To represent the wide range of experiences and histories of the Chinese ethnics in the Bay Area, I will use the term "Chinese diaspora"[8] interchangeably with "Chinese ethnic community."

From the census records of 1990 to 2008, we see a steady increase of Asian-Pacific Islander Americans in the Bay Area, from 15 percent for all counties in 1990 to 36 percent for all counties in 2008; conversely, the White population dropped from 61 percent in 1990 to 52 percent in 2008 (see Appendix, Table 1).[9]

Although the census numbers include all Asian-Pacific Islander ethnic groups, the mere visibility of the rapid growth of Asian Pacific Islander population in the area has had a real impact on the local political and even everyday power dynamics. Not only has the Asian Pacific Islander population been the second largest race group in the area for the past decade, the further diversifying of the general population is also reflected by significant decrease in the Caucasian population. The result is a Chinese ethnic population that, especially with the financially and socially equipped sector of it, is quickly catching up with, if not on equal footing with, high ranks of the political and economic hierarchy. In turn, we have here a Chinese ethnic community that has more say in "the rules of the game" compared to other parts of the country, where Caucasian or other ethnic populations dominate.

In the Bay Area, where the Chinese ethnic community is not only strong in head count but also in economy and politics, I argue it is a largely fair game in terms of power relations between the Chinese and non-Chinese sectors within the TCM practitioner community. What I mean by fair game is not in the sense of affirmative action, where everyone, regardless of ethnicity and languages spoken, is provided with the same access to the same resources. Fair game here means that, in a competitive market, the strong Chinese ethnic community, with local and transnational connections, provides individual Chinese ethnic practitioners with not only authority and confidence to define TCM theoretically and clinically, but also the proper training to exercise effective healing. On the other hand, the non-Chinese practitioners are also provided with a wide variety of local and overseas training, where they are equipped with powerful clinical tools to best meet the needs of the patients. The accesses are not the same, but the wide range of accessible resources offers practitioners abundant tools to build successful practices and businesses. And indeed, prosperous TCM practices have been built in the Bay Area by practitioners across ethnicities.

STATISTICAL DATA ON TCM PRACTITIONERS IN CALIFORNIA

In November 2006, I mailed a survey to 500 individuals across California who placed advertisements on a public online phone directory, *yellowpages.com*, under the category of "Acupuncture and Traditional Chinese Medicine."[10] One hundred and thirty eight of these practitioners responded to the survey (about a third of them were located in the Bay Area), a sample population that provides some concrete statistical groundwork for our understanding of TCM practitioners in California.[11] In the survey I focused on three aspects of the practitioners' identities: 1) their demographic location, including educational and professional credentials; 2) the presentations of their own persons and clinics, and also how they wish to be perceived by the patients/clients; and 3) their religious and/or spiritual identities, if they had regular "cultivation practices" that may impact the efficacy of their clinical practices, and if they practice energetic/spiritual healing in the clinical setting. This survey was a pilot study for this book project, and its findings helped me frame the direction of the ethnographic fieldwork that I later conducted in the Bay Area, and provides a more macro-level perspective to the TCM practitioners as a community. I will sometimes refer to these survey results in the next few chapters as supplemental data to help explain and further substantiate my field findings in the Bay Area.

Demographics

Studies on TCM practitioners in the United States have found that the practitioners are predominantly of European Caucasian and East Asian descent.[12] The TCM practitioners who responded to my survey show the same pattern: the profession is dominated by those of Caucasian descent (41 percent) and of Chinese descent (44 percent). Another 10 percent were of Korean and other Asian descents, and the remainder were the few with Latino, African, or mixed descents (see Appendix, Table 2).

My survey results also show a gender breakdown that is similar to previous studies, where there are slightly more female practitioners (52 percent) than male (40 percent). However, the 8 percent nonresponse rate for this particular item creates a grey area large enough to raise questions about whether there is a statistically significant percentage difference between genders (see Appendix, Table 3).

In terms of age group, 54 percent of my survey respondents fall squarely within the baby boomer bracket (born between 1945 and 1964); 71 percent of the respondents are between 35 and 61 years of age; and only 5 percent of the respondents are under 34 years of age. The dominance of baby boomers in the profession seems to correlate with a heightened awareness in health and health-related issues in the particular age group (see Appendix, Table 4).[13]

It is also significant to note that the majority of TCM practitioners in California come from non-medical trainings and careers; 41 percent of my informants actually have a masters or higher-level degree outside of the TCM educational system (see Appendix, Table 5).

Religiosity, Spirituality, and Practice

It is often argued, at least by the scholars in new religious movements in the United States, that the Americans are increasingly "Spiritual but not Religious,"[14] where the churchgoing "religious" are now replaced by the path-seeking "spiritual." My survey respondents seem to suggest a different model: religiosity and spirituality could be two different dimensions in life, rather than being different modes of one dimension.

In my survey, I asked the TCM practitioners to provide their religious identity or affiliation both of their upbringing and now. It is interesting to see that there was a slight drop in the number of respondents who have no religious identity or affiliation (see Appendix, Table 8); 14 percent of the respondents say they religiously identified with God in their upbringing, but now only 4 percent still do. And while those who used to identify as Christian (36 percent) have reduced in number today (19 percent), the number of Buddhists doubled (7 percent in upbringing, 14 percent now). There is also more variety in the religious identities and affiliations (see Appendix, Table 8). Perhaps this can be interpreted as a trend of going only slightly less conventional (moving from Christianity to other religions, such as Buddhism), but still staying in the safety zone of mainstream religious sensitivities (recognized institutional religions).

Now, in order to measure how "spiritual"[15] the TCM practitioners are, I tried to assess by asking the respondents about their personal "practices." I listed practices that are commonly known as "cultivation practices," where the shared goal of the activities is to cultivate the person, whether it is physically, emotionally, psychologically, or spiritually.

The variety of cultivation-type practices did not stop with my short list; respondents listed many more. Without using the term "cultivation," the respondents seem to have a relatively clear idea that "practices" here mean those exercises where one makes connections between the physical and the spiritual, between outer and the inner, between the individual and nature, and so on. And that understanding also shows in a lot of the "Other" practices they list. Some respondents listed sports regimens, and explained that the physical exercises help them get "more in tune with their own bodies." Secular sports can possibly serve the same purpose as many of the more physically oriented cultivation practices.

In line with the usual eclectic approach of the TCM practitioners, their personal practices are also multifaceted (see Appendix, Table 9). Only 15 out of 138 respondents either did not do any of these practices or chose not to answer. The rest of the respondents checked from one to many of the items on the list as activities they regularly practice. More than half (53 percent) of the respondents said they try to get in touch with nature regularly; it is interesting to note that this is popular even with people who do not have other "practices." Sitting meditation was the next popular activity (37 percent), with *qigong* exercises (31 percent) and *taichi*[16] exercises (28 percent) to follow. I would personally combine *qigong* exercises and *taichi* exercises into one category (*taichi* as one type of *qigong*), but my respondents repeatedly insisted that a separate category must be established for *taichi*. If the top four practices on the chart seem relatively secular in nature, the next two are definitely going to break the trend. Praying to God, Allah, or the Goddess is regularly practiced by 25 percent of the respondents, while communicating with spiritual beings and forces is favored by 25 percent of the respondents. There was a clear trend of regularly practicing to become more in tune with the environment, the cosmos, and within oneself; in other words, we can safely say that the TCM practitioners are doing a fair amount of spiritual cultivation in their private time (see Appendix, Table 9).

When asked how relevant the above personal practices are to their clinical practices, only 10 percent of the respondents reported they are not relevant; 72 percent of the respondents reported that these practices are either very helpful or extremely important to their clinical practices (see Appendix, Table 10). I do not therefore conclude that TCM practitioners all practice spiritual healing in their clinics. Rather, I understand the responses as demonstrating that there is significant spiritual cultivation behind their seemingly secular clinic behaviors. Also, these spiritual cultivations are not necessarily the equivalent of, or linked to, their religious identities or religiosity.

Clinical Practices

The way TCM is practiced in California very often consists of ritual-like experiences for the patients, where "ritual" can be defined as transformative activities performed in specially demarcated spaces.[17] The transformations are believed to be more than relief of physical pain and discomforts. They are also emotional/psychological, and most importantly in this case, energetic transformations. Practitioners intend their patients to experience the TCM clinic as a sanctuary-like space (Caucasian practitioners lean more toward this tendency). That is an attempt to change the patients' emotional/psychological state.

In the treatment room, the practitioners further attempt to induce emotional/psychological transformations by calming the patients. Out of all 138 respondents, only 3 percent did not respond to this question, and nobody specified not having strategies to calm the patients: 89 percent of the respondents play soothing music and natural sounds during treatment, and 68 percent try to ease the patients with calming voice and attitude. Other popular strategies include using scented candles and aromatherapy (17 percent) and having the practitioner imagine or visualize calmness (21 percent). Some practitioners try to make the treatment room environment and the treatment itself as comfortable for the patients as possible (8 percent). A few say they pray and chant during treatment (2 percent), or teach the patients breathing techniques (5 percent) (see Appendix, Table 11).

Energetic healing is often used as a complementary strategy in the TCM clinics; 43 percent of my respondents say that they incorporate some use of energy or *qi* in their clinical practices. The practitioners incorporate energetic strategies and use their senses and mental intentions to enhance the efficacy of their manual treatments. With the energy/*qi* paradigms at work in the TCM framework, a patient in treatment is transformed energetically by the practitioner by the following techniques: sensing the movements of *qi* (47 percent), attempting to move *qi* around by visualization, imagination, or intention (24 percent), or by actual *qi* or energy transfer (5 percent) (see Appendix, Table 12).

Although the energy paradigm is popular among TCM practitioners of all ethnicities, there is a wide range of understanding in how or whether "energetic" bodily experiences relate to spirituality and/or religiosity. This is a topic I will investigate more comprehensively in the next few chapters. The categories of energy sensations, altered psychological states, and spiritual experiences are defined differently across cultures, and the boundaries are also drawn differently in each sociocultural scenario. It is within the ambiguous grey areas where we can see the power dynamics between a community and the various forces that attempt to define, confine, and regulate healing practices. In these grey areas we see the TCM practitioners as a community struggling to define what they know, what they believe in, and what their role is.

My Californian respondents understand causes of diseases with categories that are predominantly of mainline holistic medicine and biomedicine; Chinese medical etiology is recognized and used, but seems to only take a secondary or complementary place in the respondents' explanations of diseases. The dominating biomedical framework and the categorization of TCM as one branch of holistic medicine have further implications in how TCM practitioners attempt to create professional images for themselves and for their clinical practices.

As an "alternative" medicine, TCM is often dichotomized and set over against biomedicine. In turn, TCM practitioners construct professional images based on a culturally accepted and understood set of elements that is regarded as positive from the biomedical standard. The practitioners then attempt to negotiate and secure their professional niche by providing more comprehensive services in the same clinic, and by creating transformative clinic spaces that provide an additional experiential dimension to the treatments.

The Californian TCM practitioners' frequent emphasis on the experiential component in their healing practices raises questions about how expressions that have common connotations of "religious" or "spiritual" are understood when they are used to describe and explain bodily experiences within the medical setting. I approach the religious/spiritual dimension within the TCM practices from three aspects: 1) the practitioners' self-identified religious affiliations; 2) whether the practitioners have personal practices that are commonly considered related to spiritual cultivation, and whether they associate those practices with the efficacy of their clinical treatments; and 3) whether they engage in spiritual-oriented activities as part of their clinical practices. The findings show that about 78 percent of the respondents identify with specific religious affiliations, and most of those affiliations are with established religions; they are more actively "religious" than the hypothesized "spiritual but not religious." The majority of TCM practitioners, even some of those who do not identify as being religiously affiliated, have practices that are commonly conceptualized as spiritual cultivation. Even more significant is the fact that 72 percent of the respondents make positive connections between the personal cultivation practices and the efficacy of their clinical treatments. Finally, it is very common among the practitioners to engage in the creation of experiences of transformation and utilization of religious/spiritually related strategies as part of their treatment routines.

TCM PRACTITIONERS IN THE BAY AREA

Out of the more than 13,000 acupuncturists licensed by the state of California, 2,855 (almost one-fifth) are located in the ten counties of the San Francisco Bay Area. The counties of Alameda, San Francisco, and Santa Clara, where there are the highest percentages of Chinese Americans, have the highest number of licensed acupuncturists as well (see Appendix, Table 13). The majority of my interview informants are also located in these three counties.

Considering practitioners in the Bay Area as a subset of practitioners in California, where practitioners in the Bay Area were also included in my California-wide survey, I assume that the statistics gathered from my survey should be fairly consistent with practitioners in the Bay Area. Although not all TCM practitioners in the Bay Area are licensed acupuncturists, the majority of my informants, even if they do not use acupuncture as their main healing modality, are licensed in acupuncture. Licensure is viewed as economically favorable for most practitioners, except for very few "niche" practitioners who have highly specialized clientele, because acupuncture is the only modality that is covered by most public and private health insurance. Even more importantly, as the only state-regulated modality in the wide array of TCM modalities, acupuncture licensing provides protection for the practitioners and the patients via eligibility for malpractice insurance. With California's acupuncture licensing exams now offered in Chinese (also in English and Korean), even those Chinese ethnic practitioners who practice in the backs of gift shops in Chinatown are mostly licensed. Therefore, it is reasonable to assume that the California State Acupuncture Board count for acupuncture licensees represents a relatively accurate estimate of all TCM practitioners in the Bay Area.

In the next few chapters, we learn about how the TCM profession has evolved in the Bay Area, how the practitioners are trained, and how they conceptualize their practices.

NOTES

1. National median on single-family house at the end of 2008 fourth quarter: $180,100; for the same period, San Francisco-Oakland-Fremont region median was $487,100, and San Jose-Sunnyvale-Santa Clara median was $525,000, both figures are results of already almost 40 percent decline from the previous quarter. See: "Metropolitan Area Existing-Home Prices and State Existing-Home Sales: Single Family Home, 2008 4th Quarter"; http://www.realtor.org/wps/wcm/connect/a0a78e804d0074afa729ef8d0a12d865/REL08Q4T.pdf?MOD=AJPERES&CACHEID=a0a78e804d0074afa729ef8d0a12d865 (accessed November 14, 2009).

2. Derived from U.S. Census dataset, searchable through U.S. Census website, American FactFinder: Fact Sheet for a Race, Ethnic, or Ancestry Group; http://factfinder.census.gov/home/saff/main.html (accessed November 14, 2009). The search was for Chinese ethnics in ten counties of the Bay Area.

3. U.S. Cenus, American FactFinder: Fact Sheet for a Race, Ethnic, or Ancestry Group.
4. See Hsiang-Shui Chen, *Chinatown No More: Taiwan Immigrants in Contemporary New York* (Ithaca, NY: Cornell University Press, 1992). From studying new Chinese immigrants in New York City, Chen realized that his Chinese informants identify themselves by class.
5. See Joe Chung Fong, "Mecca of Chinese American in California: Dai Fow (San Francisco), Yee Fow (Sacramento), and Sam Fow (Stockton)," in *150 Years of the Chinese Presence in California (1848–2001): Honor the Past, Engage the Present, Build the Future* (Sacramento, CA: Sacramento Chinese Culture Foundation; Asian American Studies, University of California, Davis, 2001); 166–67.
6. Peter Kwong, *The New Chinatown* (New York: Hill and Wang, 1996), 5; bold in original.
7. Peter Kwong, *The New Chinatown*, 5.
8. The term "diaspora" was originally used to label those communities that left and lost their homelands. If one were to look up the word "diaspora" in the American English dictionaries, one finds it first as Diaspora, with the capital D, meaning specifically the dispersed Jewish communities. Historically known as *The* Diaspora, it is reasonable to consider the Jewish Diaspora as the classic prototype for other diasporas. The Diasporans scattered geographically but maintained the traditions and customs of their extinct homeland. They were permanent refugees belonging and owning no actual geographic location until the founding of the State of Israel in 1948. Summarizing Khachig Tölöyan's description of the classic diasporas, the Diasporans were stateless and powerless, with a constant tone of lamentation. Other classic diasporas with similar historical experiences were the Armenians and the Persians.
Western colonialism and the accelerated growth of global economy created a different strand of diasporas in the past 150 years. To understand these newer diasporas, Tölöyan observes some common elements in the scholarly definitions: that the diasporic communities emigrated due to coercion; that they are believed to have clearly delimited and homogenic identities in the home country; that they actively maintain a collective memory; that they guard their boundaries; that they regard diasporans with same origins as kin; and that they maintain contact with their homelands. See Khachig Tölöyan, "Rethinking Diaspora(s): Stateless Power in the Transnational Moment," *Diaspora* 5, no. 1 (1996): 3–36.
9. Derived from U.S. Census datasets: Population Estimates for Counties by Age, Race, Sex, and Hispanic Origin: Annual Time Series: July 1, 1990 to July 1, 1999 (CO-99-12), see http://www.census.gov/popest/archives/1990s/co-99-12/casrh06.txt); Profile of General Demographic Characteristics: 2000 (DP1, see http://censtats.census.gov/data/US/01000.pdf); Annual Estimates of the Resident Population by Sex, Race, and Hispanic Origin for Counties in [STATE]: April 1, 2000 to July 1, 2008 (CC-EST2008-6RACE-[ST-FIPS], see http://www.census.gov/popest/counties/asrh/CC-EST2008-RACE6.html); Annual Estimates of the Resident Population by Sex, Race Alone or in Combination, and Hispanic Origin for Counties in [STATE]: April 1, 2000 to July 1, 2008 (CC-EST2008-5RACE-[ST-FIPS], see http://www.census.gov/popest/counties/asrh/CC-EST2008-RACE5.html) (all last accessed November 14, 2009).
10. The selection of these survey recipients was random. I mailed the survey to the first 500 listings (some listed by clinic names and some by practitioner names) that provided a clear contact address that I could mail to. Some initial mailings were not successfully delivered (perhaps the practices had moved), and I went further down the listing until five hundred surveys were successfully received, meaning that they were not returned to sender via the post office.
11. Please note that this particular survey included practitioners across the entire state and far beyond the geographic framing of this book; the results had informed my later fieldwork in the Bay Area, and is a helpful set of information for contextualizing my ethnographic findings in the Bay Area. Although some of the practitioners who answered the survey were located in the Bay Area, the overall statistics should not be

taken as equivalent and representative of the perspectives and positions of Bay Area practitioners.

12. Martha Hare, "The Emergence of an Urban U.S. Chinese Medicine," *Medical Anthropology Quarterly* 1, no. 1 (1993); Karen Okicich et al., *Acupuncture Practice* (Office of Examination Resources, California Department of Consumer Affairs, 2001).

13. See Jan A. English-Lueck, *Health in the New Age: A Study of California Holistic Practices* (Albuquerque: University of New Mexico Press, 1990); Robert C. Fuller, *Spiritual, but Not Religious: Understanding Unchurched America* (Oxford; New York: Oxford University Press, 2001); Kimberly J. Lau, *New Age Capitalism: Making Money East of Eden* (Philadelphia: University of Pennsylvania Press, 2000).

14. See Fuller, *Spiritual, but Not Religious: Understanding Unchurched America*; also Robert Wuthnow, *After Heaven: Spirituality in America since the 1950s* (Berkeley; Los Angeles; London: University of California Press, 1998).

15. I use this term in the most general sense of it as the metaphysical aspect of people's experiences in life. It will actually be my goal to understand how my informants understand and define the term.

16. *Taichi* is the popularly spelling for *taiji* 太極 in the American mainstream. It is a form of martial art or moving meditation that the Chinese commonly identify as *taijiquan*太極拳.

17. In Victor Turner's sense of "ritual." See Victor Turner, "Symbol, Myth, and Ritual," in *The Ritual Process: Structure and Anti-Structure*, ed. Victor Turner (Ithaca: Cornell University Press, 1969), 95.

TWO
Evolution of TCM in the Bay Area

In Truckee, a small, historically frontier town in Northern California, stands a Chinese herbal shop that dates back to 1878. This small brick building is the sole remnant of the third Chinatown that the Chinese American community built in Truckee in the 1870s.[1] Archaeological studies on San Jose's historic Heinlenville Chinatown, constructed in 1887 and demolished in 1932, also identified records and remains of medicinal herb shops.[2] At the height of Anti-Chinese sentiment and enforcement of the Chinese Exclusion Act (1882), the White community aggressively destroyed Chinatowns across Northern California by repeatedly setting fires. Chinese American communities responded by moving and rebuilding their homes and businesses, supporting one another and with the help of the few sympathetic White neighbors. As part of the tireless efforts of building and rebuilding, herbal shops and traditional Chinese healers were always crucial components in the Chinatowns in Northern California since the early days of Chinese immigration.

Little is known about those individuals who cared for the medical needs of the Chinatown residents in the era of active Chinese Exclusion. These healers served the Chinese American communities without leaving much in the way of official documentation or personal records. Photo documentation of significant moments of Chinese American history in the Bay Area show proud records of individuals who became Western biomedical doctors, the perceived epitome of successful integration into mainstream America.[3] In contrast, traditional Chinese doctors in Chinatowns were largely silent and invisible, at least in terms of historic documentation. But they definitely did exist, and were probably instrumental in providing healthcare to Chinese American communities, especially in eras when White society was decidedly hostile toward Chinese Americans.

From the mainstream American perspective, President Richard Nixon's visit to China in 1972 marked a new era for traditional Chinese medicine. The opening of China and the ensuing diplomatic relationship between China and the United States brought new attention to China as a rising new ally, and to Chinese acupuncture as the exciting new medical "discovery." With attention from the mainstream media, traditional Chinese medicine finally escaped the confines of Chinatowns and entered the consciousness of mainstream American society.

Acupuncture became the primary modality in traditional Chinese medicine outside of the Chinese societies and Chinese ethnic communities in the United States for several reasons. First is the fact that acupuncture as a modality is used in several medical systems: Japanese, Korean, and Vietnamese traditional medicines all use acupuncture, with their own medical theories and techniques, and there have also been French (via Indo-China) and American style acupuncture derived from these traditional systems. Not all acupuncturists who practice in California practice Chinese acupuncture; however, the California licensing exam for acupuncture is based entirely on the TCM system. The domination of TCM over other Asian traditional medical systems in California through the licensing of a shared modality deserves its own separate research project. The bottom line: while many non-Chinese acupuncturists encounter the modality through non-Chinese medical systems, by licensing acupuncture with exclusively Chinese medical theories, TCM in turn extends its turf significantly through the licensed modality.

The second reason acupuncture became the trophy modality in TCM in America traces back to two specific historical moments. Journalist James Reston's 1971 article in *The New York Times* recounting his experience undergoing an appendectomy in Beijing (previously Romanized as Peking), where he received acupuncture for post-surgery pain management, first stirred attention toward acupuncture in the American mainstream consciousness.[4] Later, Reston was often mis-referenced as having undergone acupuncture anesthesia for the surgery, which is completely untrue. In the article itself, Reston specifies that he had undergone a standard biomedical surgery with "normal injection of Xylocain and Benzocain, which anesthetized the middle of [his] body."[5] Nonetheless, the possibility of using a few needles in place of expensive narcotic to anesthetize wildly sparked the imaginations of the American public: What else can those little needles do that biomedicine cannot?

Another significant historical moment contributing to the fame of acupuncture happened in the state of Nevada. In 1973, Nevada became the first state in the United States to legalize acupuncture, herbs, and other Chinese healing practices. Although California and New York had longer histories of traditional Chinese medicine being practiced and a substantial number of practitioners, the key to bringing traditional Chinese medicine onto the Nevada lawmakers' agenda was an acupuncture clinic which opened across the street from the state house for two weeks with special permission from the state senate.[6]

A New York lawyer and real estate tycoon by the name of Arthur Steinberg was behind this effort, which took him several years of hard selling, financial investment, and strategic politicking. On a trip to Asia in 1972, Steinberg and his wife, Mia, encountered an acupuncturist in Hong Kong who cured Mia's migraines, which had tortured her for many years. Steinberg recorded his wife's treatments on film, and upon his return to the United States, founded the American Society of Acupuncture to promote the practice. He first approached the biomedical community to seek its support and endorsement, but the reactions were lukewarm at best. Undeterred, Steinberg invited Lok Yee Kung 陸易公, the acupuncturist who cured his wife in Hong Kong, to Nevada. The Nevada Medical Board unanimously voted against giving Lok temporary permission to practice.

Disappointed by the lack of support from the medical community, Steinberg decided to go to the public. He bought time on television to talk about acupuncture, and urged the viewers to call their legislative representatives to allow practice of the effective healing modality. Simultaneously, Steinberg's lobbyist approached the lawmakers individually in the attempt to gain their support. After arranging for Lok to perform privately on several members of the House of Representatives and state senate, an emergency amendment passed both houses and was signed by the governor to overturn the decision by the State Medical Board. The amendment issued special permission for Lok to practice for two weeks to demonstrate his medical art.

The by now much publicized demonstrations attracted public and media attention, and Steinberg's team made sure that the volunteer patients included not only persons from the public but also journalists and more lawmakers. By the end of the two weeks, while patients continued to flow into the temporary clinic across the street to seek acupuncture treatments, the lawmakers had legalized traditional Chinese medicine as "a learned profession."[7] The legal breakthrough prompted other states to follow suit. Interestingly, there had been preciously few practicing acupuncturists in Nevada. As of August 23, 2009, the Nevada State Board of Oriental Medicine lists only forty-five active licensees for the entire state.[8]

These two historical moments, one commonly mis-referenced and the other mostly forgotten, became seeds of the eventual flourishing of acupuncture as the model modality of traditional Chinese medicine in the United States. The image of just a few small needles inserted in various parts of the body became an iconic contrast to biomedicine's increasing reliance on complicated machines and expensive laboratory tests, and the early testimonies of effective treatments often consisted of miraculous cures of health problems that biomedicine had failed to treat effectively.

Furthermore, the comparatively low cost of TCM treatments allowed practitioners to provide services to underprivileged populations. In other words, traditional Chinese medicine became a complementary medicine that filled much of the void in biomedicine, not only in terms of medical strategies but also in reaching certain neglected socioeconomic sectors. Spiritual orientations aside, some practitioners started their journey in the profession to help provide more comprehensive healthcare right in the biomedical framework.

FOUR PHASES OF TCM IN THE BAY AREA

In the following, I will trace the development of traditional Chinese medicine in the Bay Area through the lives and narratives of four licensed acupuncturists, who represent important (and sometimes overlapping) phases in the local history of traditional Chinese medicine. The legend of Miriam Lee, a respected pioneer practitioner who was known for her political activism, represents a generation of acupuncturists who established a political foundation that gradually led legal sanction of acupuncture in California. Sophia tells of a journey that resonates with the path of those acupuncturists who resisted the impersonal approach of biomedicine and promoted a self-reflective, patient-centered, humanistic interpretation of the practices. Crystal recalls the history of AIDS epidemic in San Francisco, where, through selfless service and social engagement, acupuncturists gradually became part of the general healthcare community in the city. Finally, Jason shares his story on the continuing efforts by acupuncturists to enhance their professional image. Perhaps as a reflection of how the different phases of this history relate to each other, although not forming an official lineage, Miriam Lee served as a mentor for all three other acupuncturists included in this chapter.

Political Foundation: Miriam Lee

Miriam Lee (Chinese name: Li Chuan-zhen 李傳真), dubbed by some local practitioners and patients as "Mother of Acupuncture in California," was probably one of the first practitioners of traditional Chinese medicine who came into the American mainstream public eye. The now-deceased pioneer was best known for being arrested for practicing medicine without a license in 1974; the incident ended with her release a few days later after over a hundred of her patients, both Chinese and Caucasian, showed up at the courthouse in protest of her arrest and requested her release.[9] The dramatic incident, along with the petitions and negotiations of many other pioneer acupuncturists, their patients, and sympathizers, prompted the eventual certification and licensing of acupuncture in California.[10]

In coalition with other practitioners, Miriam went on to actively advocate for broadening the scope of practice for certified acupuncturists, and the eventual licensing of the profession. She founded the Acupuncture Association of America (AAA) in 1980, which provided continuing education courses in acupuncture and attempted to exert political influence. For $1,000 a month, coming out of Miriam's own pocket (she charged $20 per acupuncture treatment), she hired lobbyist Art Krause to draft and promote bill proposals with key legislators in Sacramento. In 1989, Miriam also helped found the Council of Acupuncture Organizations to facilitate cooperation between the several acupuncture associations in California.

The daughter of Chinese Christian missionaries, Miriam was born and raised in Shandong province, China, and trained in Western biomedicine as a nurse and midwife. In 1949 she left China for Singapore, and lived there for seventeen years before moving to the United States.[11] Her students are not consistent about when she learned acupuncture or where she learned it,[12] but by the time she came to the Bay Area in the 1960s, she worked in the factory assembly line at Hewlett-Packard during the day, and practiced acupuncture after work.[13]

By the early 1970s, Miriam already had a busy full-time acupuncture practice in Palo Alto, California. In the early days of her practice, when there were very few traditional Chinese doctors in the Peninsula region, her students recalled that she saw eighty to a hundred patients a day. The Chinese who lived in the area came to her, but Miriam also had a very strong Caucasian patient base. Furthermore, in the era when there were not yet any schools of traditional Chinese medicine in California, Miriam was responsible for training many of the first generation of Caucasian acupuncturists in the Bay Area.[14] She and her clinic continued to serve as an important education center for the Bay Area acupuncturists even after the acupuncture schools were established. Her clinic accepted graduates from local acupuncture schools as interns, and invited famous acupuncturists from around the United States and abroad to teach continuing education courses to practicing acupuncturists.

After retirement, Miriam moved to the Los Angeles area to reside with her family until her death in 2009. She never married and had no children. Her student Susan Johnson inherited AAA, which still operates out of Santa Cruz today.

Humanistic Interpretation: Sophia[15]

Sophia practices in a house in a quiet residential area. The carpeted interior is slightly dated, creating a welcoming atmosphere much like many of the first-generation Chinese American houses I have visited. Sophia is in her fifties, casually dressed, with the warmth that reminds me of my own mother and aunts. Soon I learned that she is a philosopher by training. An immigrant from Taiwan, she is the prodigy of Mou Zongsan 牟宗三, one of the most recognized Chinese Kantian (after Immanuel Kant) philosophers. In fact, she has written and published a collection of essays in Chinese that includes two chapters on a Kantian approach to understanding traditional Chinese medicine in the United States. When I first interviewed her in 2008, she was still teaching and practicing traditional Chinese medicine, but was planning to decrease her acupuncture workload and focus more on philosophy. By 2009, she has almost completely shifted to full-time work on her philosophical writings.

Sophia's entry into traditional medicine was unintentional. In 1977, Sophia took a leave of absence from her graduate studies in philosophy at a prestigious university in Taiwan to immigrate to the Unites States with her husband. To help support the household, she found a job working in a traditional Chinese clinic. The woman who ran the clinic was Miriam Lee.

Miriam already had many interns working in the clinic at the time. Sophia had no previous training in traditional Chinese medicine, but found it fascinating to observe the clinical practices. She also realized that the theories behind the practices were intrinsically related to natural philosophy. Already an avid reader, she began to collect classical texts on Chinese medicine whenever she travelled back to Taiwan. At first she studied for fun, and never thought she would pursue a real career in Chinese medicine.

In the early 1980s, Miriam started to invite experienced practitioners to her clinic to provide monthly continuing education classes to her students and other practitioners in the Bay Area. It was also during this time that Sophia engaged herself more seriously in traditional Chinese medicine. She learned from Miriam in the day-to-day clinic practices, and rubbed shoulders with famous practitioners invited from China and Taiwan.

Sophia eventually went back to Taiwan to obtain her masters degree in philosophy. After that, she returned to the Bay Area, and started to practice acupuncture professionally in 1987. Like many experienced acupuncturists in the Bay Area, she trained interns in her clinic, consistent with the tradition of apprenticeship in the traditional Chinese medical practices.

Although Sophia does not self-identify as a Confucian elite (contemporary Chinese scholars rarely do), she communicates some of Confucianism's central values: she emphasizes the medical classics as the root of knowledge, and she embodies critically self-reflective understanding of healing as a humanistic and ongoing practice. Sophia is also aware of the shifting between her role as a healer and as a teacher:

> When people come in as my patients, the way I treat them is different. They have all my focus. But it comes to study or teaching with demon-

stration, the priority shifts to the students, or whatever observers, say when you are around. My obligation will shift to you guys. I would treat the patient more like an object. And some people are okay with this, but some people are not. When I practice with just the patient, I listen to them, their issues, the process of the knowledge is in my mind, I don't have to lay it out. I have no obligation to any student [when there are no interns around].

She further explains:

In the very traditional way of apprenticeship, you are not supposed to talk. You just observe. All the talking . . . I try not to talk in front of patients. Because we get excited about difficult cases, and we forget about the person who is suffering. We really try to treat patients as patients, as subjects, as human beings.

In the 1990s, Miriam took a hiatus for two years for health reasons. Sophia was asked to take over Miriam's practice in Palo Alto. With her own practice in the South Bay, she travelled between the two clinics and took care of Miriam's patients while Miriam was away. In turn, she continued the mission of educating patients and acupuncturists not only in her own practice but also in Miriam's practice. Especially when there were not yet any accredited acupuncture schools in the South Bay,[16] Sophia served as a mentor for many acupuncture interns who lived in the area.

Besides promoting the patient-centered approach, Sophia also represents a more classical perspective in the profession, while the acupuncture schools systematically imported the "scientific" Chinese medicine to its students through China-trained practitioners who mostly aimed to justify the medicine with scientific evidence, and specifically with biomedicine. However, there seems to be increasing appreciation in perspectives like Sophia's. Several acupuncturists I interviewed describe traditional Chinese medicine more as a craft or art rather than merely a medical modality, and say that they are just beginning to seek inspirations from classical texts.[17] In fact, local acupuncture programs are increasingly recognizing the importance of medical classics in the training of new acupuncturists. A decade ago, only one of the four local acupuncture programs required courses in Chinese medical classics; currently, all the acupuncture schools in the Bay Area require at least one course in Chinese medical classics for graduation.

Social Engagement: Crystal[18]

Although sometimes considered less authentic compared to Chinese ethnic practitioners, traditional Chinese medicine practiced by Caucasian Americans enabled the crossing of ethnic boundaries and reached some populations that have very little contact or exposure to Chinese people and the Chinese culture in general. Largely through Caucasian practitioners with backgrounds and connections in biomedicine networks, acupuncturists as a group began to reach skeptical biomedical doctors across ethnic and cultural barriers.

Crystal belongs to the earliest group of Bay Area acupuncturists who were trained by the local acupuncture schools. After finishing her course work, Crystal interned with Miriam Lee, who became her mentor and role model.

In the early 1980s, the AIDS epidemic was sweeping through the gay community in the city of San Francisco. The biomedical health providers were confronted with the reality of this new and mysterious infection taking their patients' lives. Some AIDS patients sought alternative healings outside of biomedicine, and found their way to the acupuncturists. Probably out of both compassion toward the patients and desperation due to the lack of a cure, some biomedical hospitals in the area allowed acupuncturists to treat their AIDS patients right in the hospital rooms when necessary.

It was not easy working in such an intense environment with the deadly disease, especially for a new practitioner who was still working on honing her clinical skills:

> In the beginning, when I first realized that I just contacted HIV . . . I mean, I didn't contract it, but here is this patient sitting with me, we don't know how it's contracted. I cried all the way home. But at the same time, it also made sense to recognize that the health practitioners were not dropping like flies. People were dying from direct contact that could be identified. The health practitioners who were coming down with the virus were people who had blood squirted into their eye or a needle had jumped from a patient and to them. Something had happened.

Crystal and her acupuncturist peers were fearful of the new disease, but also optimistic, especially after seeing positive results from their treatments on the patients. The acupuncturists could not cure AIDS. However, they helped prolong lives of some of the patients, and helped others improve the quality of their lives especially in the last days of their lives. Acupuncture treatments were so helpful that Crystal was able to establish her first practice in San Francisco treating mostly AIDS patients.

The epidemic crisis created a type of acupuncture clinic in San Francisco that provided not just medical treatment, but also a place where the patients supported one another:

> We had two big rooms with French doors in between them, and what wound up happening was that the patients all decided to open the French doors and all four people got treated together, like one room. Like a family situation. And we cared about each other. They laughed with each other. They would all come in at the same general time each

week, so they got to know the people who were at the tables while they were there.

The above-mentioned new model was one of the first community clinics in the Bay Area. Community clinics, a unique form of acupuncture clinic that is seen mostly in the cities of San Francisco and Berkeley, do more than just serve the nearby community and provide care to underprivileged populations. The clinic offers a space where the patients actually form a community of mutual support while they undergo treatments. The acupuncture schools in San Francisco and Berkeley now offer this type of clinic as a way to provide acupuncture treatments at almost no cost to the patients, and the students benefit from having more patients with whom they can practice their skills

At the same time that she established the AIDS clinic in San Francisco, Crystal also had another practice in Santa Cruz, a liberal college town by the coast, where she had been living. Unlike the city of San Francisco, Santa Cruz has always had a very small Chinese ethnic population. On the other hand, the University of California in Santa Cruz maintains fresh rotations of diverse student populations from out-of-town and out-of-state. The predominantly Caucasian population of Santa Cruz was open-minded, but nowhere close to the progressive and free-spirited San Franciscans.

In Santa Cruz, Crystal found herself in another niche. Although intended to be a general practice, 80 percent of Crystal's patients were abuse victims at one point. Mostly women, these patients came to her with physical complaints, but Crystal found that often their physical conditions were linked to experiences of abuse and emotional trauma. Combining her skills in traditional Chinese medicine with her previous training in psychotherapy and guided meditation, she helped her patients heal their bodies, minds, and spirits.

Crystal ended her practice in San Francisco after a few years of grueling commutes from Santa Cruz, but her Santa Cruz practice has served the community for more than thirty years now. Currently, her practice is a general family practice where she cares for families of patients, sometimes even their pets. She has seen her baby patients grow into adulthood, and they bring their babies back to her clinic. It is not a community clinic in the sense of an open clinic, but it provides care for the community that meets the needs of a wide range of patients through different stages of their lives.

Although Crystal does not speak Chinese and has not been closely associated with the Chinese ethnic community, she is acquainted with some of the pioneer practitioners in Chinatown and speaks of them respectfully. After Miriam retired, Crystal continued her mentor's mission to educate her fellow practitioners by teaching workshops around the country.

Identity Enhancement: Jason[19]

This fourth phase of development in traditional Chinese medicine in the Bay Area came as a result of the influx of immigrants from People's Republic of China (PRC) starting in the late 1990s—among the new immigrants were some of the most talented and experienced practitioners of traditional Chinese medicine from PRC. Some of these immigrant practitioners are hired by the Bay Area acupuncture schools to educate local students. Others find themselves acquiring a California license for acupuncture and establishing clinics in their new homeland.

In his forties but looking more like in his early thirties, Jason is soft-spoken yet extremely confident, and combines suaveness with sincerity in just the perfect proportions. He grew up in a rural farming village in the Liaoning province in China, and became a barefoot doctor when he was very young. Later he worked his way to medical school and specialized in acupuncture, neurology, and sports medicine.

In 1996, Jason was invited to teach a seminar for the acupuncturists in the Bay Area. After the lively seminar, one female acupuncturist pulled him to the side and said, "You know, I have never met a doctor from China who didn't require a translator. You are the first. You are young and speak great English, why don't you move here to practice? We need a good Chinese doctor like you."

That woman was Miriam Lee. She put her words into action: with her connections, one of the acupuncture schools hired Jason to teach, which granted him a working visa and ticket to America. For the first two years, Jason worked in Miriam's clinic on days off from his teaching job. Quickly, he accumulated enough financial capital and patient base to start his own clinic. His business was a success. Not only does he now own the property where his clinic is situated, he plans to open three more clinics and hire some of his students to practice in them.

By the time Jason immigrated to the Bay Area, acupuncture was already licensed and recognized with an impressive scope of practice. On the other hand, acupuncturists are still not considered "physicians," and although health insurance companies are required by state law to provide coverage for acupuncture treatments, the payments are significantly lower compared to payments to biomedical physicians. More and more insurance companies are paying only $25 per session, limited to twelve treatments in a calendar year. Considering that a typical acupuncture treatment can take anywhere from half an hour to two hours, it is easy to understand why some Bay Area acupuncturists are suffering financially.

Jason keenly realizes that there is still a lack of recognition for traditional Chinese medicine as an equal on the local medical hierarchy. And he sees that the problem starts from within the profession and the educational system:

> The current education for [traditional Chinese medicine in the Bay Area] is inadequate, and the image for [the practitioners] is not too good either. Everybody thinks that Chinese doctors are cheap, and acupuncture doesn't take too much time to learn. Whereas [biomedical] schools are very serious, people think of acupuncture schools in terms of this one slightly more expensive, that one slightly cheaper [in tuition]. I think there is something very wrong with that. In the [American universities], professors are on tenure track. In our [acupuncture] school, if I teach for one hour they pay me for one hour, if I don't teach then there is nothing, and there are no benefits at all. I don't like that, mostly because I don't feel respected.

The lack of respect has more to do with the dignity of the teaching profession than the actual pay. Jason tries to illustrate his point with yet more calculations:

> I tell [the school] that I demand a pay increase.... In the end, even if they pay me $120, it's really $30-40 an hour including preparation. I say, [if I want to make good money], all I have to do is sit and drink some tea in my clinic. I see two patients an hour, and my new patients get charged $180, that is $360 an hour. I deserve to be paid better when I teach at the school.

Jason believes in advancing the general impression of the traditional Chinese medical profession, starting with the demand to increase the practitioners' market value. On the other hand, what he does not talk about is how the schools are able to hire teachers with such low pay. Acupuncture schools often hire instructors from China with extremely low hourly pay in exchange for a working visa or sponsorship for permanent residency. Many practitioners from China, including Jason himself, were only able to legally reside and work in the United States through such an arrangement.

Jason further suggests that acupuncturists from China should adapt to the American market:

> [The Chinese immigrant practitioners] are not good with changes. What do you say, [in English] "When in Rome, walk like [sic] the Romans do." ... It is against the spirit (*jingshen* 精神) of Chinese medicine to use the same needles and techniques on everyone. Traditional Chinese medicine must be tailored to the person, the season, and the illness (*yinren yinshi yinbing* 因人因時因病).
> When Americans come in, they say, "I am afraid of pain," then we need to slowly lead them to the sensations of how the needling is effective. Many practitioners from China are not good at being adaptive like that.

Essentially, Jason provides a model for immigrant practitioners to assimilate or at least adjust to the host society through the lens of clinical practice.

Besides the professional setting, Jason taps into the pulse of the American society through his church. Unaffiliated with any religion when he first came, he was invited to attend a Protestant congregation in Milpitas, and eventually got baptized. Like many immigrants from China, Protestantism completes the package as part of the American cultural immersion:

> I observe in the church what people say, what they do, what they eat, and their responses to life and death. Also, I get in touch with a lot of people there. They know I'm a doctor, and they refer patients to me. Sometimes they also ask me [about their own ailments]. It expands the point of contact between me and the rest of the society.

A competitive decathlon athlete, Jason trains regularly and participates in other team sports in the community. Unlike many practitioners from China who put in extremely long hours at the clinic, Jason stresses the importance of demonstrating a healthier lifestyle to his patients:

> There are more successful practitioners than I, who see forty, fifty patients a day. They have no time to even eat, and they faint. After two, three years of this kind of life, their hair all turns grey. Or they become obese. Chinese work very hard when they put their minds to it. I tell my patients, I ask you to exercise because I am an athlete myself. I am your role model, and I can assure you that exercise is effective. I teach them how to exercise, and go to the ball court to show them what to do.

And perhaps the demonstration is also for his children, who were born and raised in the Bay Area. His ten-year-old daughter has shown great interest in his clinic work, and has been allowed to be the little helper since she was six years old. Despite her young age, Jason shares as much medical knowledge with her as she can understand. After all, apprenticeship is how medical knowledge had been passed down in many Chinese medical families throughout history. Even in the dreamland of America, the Chinese tradition carries on.

RECAP: AN EVOLVING HEALTHCARE PROFESSION IN CALIFORNIA

From practicing in the backs of cramped herb stores in Chinatown to becoming legally recognized medical professionals, practitioners of traditional Chinese medicine in the Bay Area had their fair share of struggles as the profession grew and evolved. In the 1970s, the challenge for practitioners was to establish legitimacy—not just in terms of medical efficacy, but also in terms of legal sanction for them to practice at all. Miriam Lee and some other pioneer practitioners expanded their clientele beyond the Chinese ethnic enclaves, and strategically strengthened their positions through political networking in the state capitol.

In those days when the practitioners were almost exclusively Chinese ethnics, the recognition of traditional Chinese medicine by way of acupuncture as a legally sanctioned modality was a triumph not just for the sake of the medicine but also for the entire Chinese ethnic community. No longer merely sojourners who provided physical labor and contributed little to the social or intellectual culture, the Chinese acupuncturists had reached out to contribute to the well-being of American society in general. In that process of boundary-crossing, the Chinese ethnic community also discovered useful strategies for establishing political influence in the mainstream society. Miriam Lee helped legitimate acupuncture through the power of lobbying in the state senate. Later acupuncturists also formed several associations to further ensure that their voices are recognized and their rights are protected.

Sophia's story exemplifies a second phase of the evolution of the profession in the Bay Area: besides legitimizing the technical skills in the healing, she educates her students and treats her patients with humanistic awareness, intellectual sensibility, and self-reflection. Although most teachers of traditional Chinese medicine were not trained in Western philosophy, Sophia and some other practitioners brought to the foreground the importance of cultural, linguistic, and literary knowledge in traditional medical practices. In other words, practitioners with this orientation challenge the assumption that biomedicine and the Western scientific culture behind the medicine serve as the sole and standard source of legitimate medical knowledge. Acknowledging Chinese medical and literary classics as sources of medical knowledge, Sophia and her colleagues recovered additional sources of power for legitimacy outside of the American culture and biomedical paradigm.

Crystal's sociocultural location as a Caucasian American and interests in New Age spirituality and psychology were consistent with a movement that propelled traditional Chinese medicine in the Bay Area toward yet another phase of its evolution. On the one hand, Caucasian American practitioners like Crystal introduced traditional Chinese healings and ideas to their Caucasian American clientele and more broadly to the American mainstream. At the same time, the practitioners themselves and their patients brought into the medicine their preconceptions, issues, and interpretations to make it a distinctly American version of the traditional medicine.

Throughout the 1980s and 1990s, traditional Chinese medicine gained popularity in the American mainstream and also some traction in the medical marketplace. As a licensed modality, acupuncture rose to a position of prominence among alternative and complementary medical modalities: major biomedical corporations incorporated it into their services, insurance companies offered coverage for acupuncture treatments, and acupuncture schools multiplied. The continually growing community of locally trained and licensed Caucasian American practitioners quickly became the faces and voices of traditional Chinese medicine for non-Chinese ethnic patients and mainstream media. Racist-based discriminations against traditional Chinese medicine, whether outwardly articulated or not, rapidly decreased with the growth of Caucasian practitioners.

The influx of new immigrant practitioners from China in the 1990s challenged this growing power of Caucasian American practitioners. Practitioners like Jason, who was trained by state-run medical school in China, claimed authority in the profession with their competency in Chinese language and culture, and the insistence on a proper and scientific interpretation of traditional Chinese medicine. The upward mobility of successful immigrant practitioners like Jason granted them not only financial stability but also social influence. Whereas Miriam attained media visibility by her ability to mobilize her Caucasian patients and effected political change by sponsoring a lobbyist in Sacramento, Jason advances the market worth and professional image of practitioners of traditional Chinese medicine by demanding better work conditions and higher compensation.

From the stories of these acupuncturists, we see that traditional Chinese medicine has transformed to reflect the needs of its local context. Through proactive political negotiations, tireless knowledge transmissions, inventive new clinical applications, and suave upgrading of their professional image, the practitioners not only stay in business, but more importantly, provide ever-improving healthcare to the general public.

NOTES

1. See Nancy Wey, "A History of Chinese Americans in California," *Five Views: An Ethnic Historic Site Survey for California* (1988), http://www.nps.gov/history/history/online_books/5views/5views3.htm (accessed November 14, 2009).

2. See Sonoma State University History of San Jose project, http://www.sonoma.edu/asc/projects/sanjose/Part_of_San_Jose_History.pdf (accessed November 14, 2009).

3. See Laverne Mau Dicker, *The Chinese in San Francisco: A Pictorial History* (New York: Dover Publications, 1979); Lillian Gong-Guy, *Chinese in San Jose and the Santa Clara Valley*, ed. Lillian Gong-Guy and Gerrye Wong, Chinese Historical and Cultural Project (Charleston, SC: Arcadia Publishing, 2007).

4. James Reston, "Now, Let Me Tell You About My Appendectomy in Peking," *The New York Times*, July 26, 1971.

5. James Reston, "Now, Let Me Tell You About My Appendectomy in Peking."

6. "The Nation: Acupuncture in Nevada," http://www.time.com/time/magazine/article/0,9171,945215,00.html (accessed August 23, 2009).

7. For more details on the process of Steinberg's success in getting acupuncture legalized in Nevada, see Robert Schwartz, "Acupuncture and Expertise: A Challenge to Physician Control," *The Hastings Center Report* 11, no. 2 (1981); Yongming Li, "The War between Dragon and Snake: The Birth of First Legalization of Traditional Chinese Medicine in the United States (Longshe Dazhan: Meiguo Diyige Zhongyifa De Dansheng 龍蛇大戰: 美國第一個中醫法的誕生)," *World Journal Weekend Special*, March 9, 2008.

8. See Nevada State Board of Oriental Medicine official website http://oriental.nv.gov/qry-licensees_name.asp (accessed August 23, 2009).

9. On July 15, 1974, one day before Miriam's arrest, then California governor Ronald Reagon had just signed to allow acupuncture as an "experimental procedure." See Miriam Lee, *Insights of a Senior Acupuncturist* (Boulder: Blue Poppy Press, 1992), xi.

10. In 1975, California Governor Jerry Brown signed a law to legalize acupuncture by certification (SB 86 Macone-Song), which allowed acupuncturists to practice without the supervision of an MD. By 1978 the Torres Bill (AB 1291) recognized acupuncturists as primary health providers, and no longer required prior diagnosis and referrals from MDs, dentists, podiatrists, or chiropractors. In the same year, the Keysor Bill (AB2424) authorized Medi-Cal payments for acupuncture treatments. Although not typically considered "physicians" (except within the Worker's Compensation system, where they are granted authority to diagnose and treat work-related injuries, but not to diagnose disabilities), acupuncturists in California have since been given the authority to diagnose and treat patients independently. Today, acupuncturists in California are licensed by examination administered by the Acupuncture Board, which is an autonomous body under the state Department of Consumer Affairs. For more information, see "History" on California Acupuncture Board website http://www.acupuncture.ca.gov/about_us/history.shtml (accessed October 30, 2011).

11. See Susan Johnson, "Dr. Miriam Lee" http://www.tungspoints.net/bios.php#MiriamLee (accessed November 14, 2009).

12. Some students suspect that Miriam studied with Master Tung (Dong Jing-chang 董景昌), a Shandong native who propagated his family's unique style of acupuncture as Master Tung's Magic Points (Dongshi qixue董氏奇穴), for a brief period of time when they were both in Shandong. There is no evidence to this claim. In 1987, Miriam invited Dr. Young Wei-chieh (Yang Wei-jie楊維傑), who was one of the official disciples of Master Tung in Taiwan, to a year-long residency at the Acupuncture Association of America, where he lectured and demonstrated for Miriam and her students, most notably Susan Johnson and Esther Su. Later, Miriam published *Master Tong's Acupuncture: An Ancient Alternative Style in Modern Clinical Practice* (Boulder: Blue Poppy Press, 1992), a commentated translation of Master Tung's book in Chinese. Dr. Young now practices in the Los Angeles area, and also teaches courses on Master Tung's points. Susan Johnson currently teaches courses on Master Tung's points across the country. Esther Su, although not focused on teaching as much as Susan, also had many students interning in her clinic over the years. Consequently, there seems to be a branch of acupuncturists in California coming from this unofficial lineage of Master Tung's acupuncture.

13. See Knight Ridder, "Palo Alto Acupuncture Pioneer Miriam Lee, 82, Dies," *Palo Alto Daily News*, July 1, 2009.

14. The Wikipedia entry on Miriam Lee estimates that about 70 percent of the acupuncturists practicing in Northern California in the 1970s and 1980s were Miriam's students. See Wikipedia, "Miriam Lee," accessed October 31, 2011, http://en.wikipedia.org/wiki/Miriam_Lee. It is unclear how the Wikipedia percentage was calculated, but many veteran acupuncturists I interviewed attested that Miriam was one of the most influential teachers in the area.

15. Personal interview with Sophia, April 22, 2008. The interview was conducted almost entirely in English, where she occasionally used a few terms in Chinese for accuracy.

16. All the acupuncture programs in the South Bay were established after 2000. Before that, students had to go to San Francisco, Oakland, or Santa Cruz to attend an accredited acupuncture school.

17. Personal interviews with Thomas, April 28, 2008; Alison, November 12, 2008; George, October 18, 2008; Rafael, November 7, 2008.

18. Personal interview with Crystal, February 16, 2009.

19. Personal interview with Jason, April 24, 2008. The interview was almost entirely in Mandarin Chinese, and the quotes were translated into English by the author.

THREE

Knowledge Transmission and Identity Formation of an "Alternative" Medicine

In Elizabeth Hsu's *Knowledge Transmission in Chinese Medicine*, she identifies three modes of transmission she observed in her fieldwork in China: secret transmission, personal transmission, and standardized transmission. The three modes are identified by the relationship between the practitioner teacher or master and their acolytes, apprentices, or students. Secret transmission refers to the mode when the knowledge is "intentionally made secret, and [the secrecy] is crucial for the social relationship of those involved."[1] Personal transmission, according to Hsu, is subsumed under secret transmission, for it depends on the consensus between the mentor and the student to maintain a relationship of mutual trust within which the learning takes place. Finally, the standardized mode of transmission is where the knowledge is standardized and systematized, or, as Hsu explains, generally conceptualized as being Westernized, modernized, and professionalized. The transmission of knowledge in this last mode does not depend so much on a personal relationship as the first two.

Hsu observes that these transmission modes correlate with different types of healing practices within the scope of traditional Chinese medicine in China, where the *qigong* masters adhere to secret transmission, government-run institutions provide standardized transmission, and a wide range of practitioners exercise personal transmission somewhere between the two modes. In essence, these three modes signify different levels of commitment and trust between the mentor and the student, and how that interpersonal proximity of individuals involved directly determines one's access to medical knowledge.

Volker Scheid, who frames his study based on Hsu's work, also observes in his fieldwork how personal relationships determine the level of access to knowledge. He additionally points out that in the last imperial era, Chinese society had two distinct types of physicians: the hereditary physicians (*shiyi* 世醫) who attained training through family lines, and the literati physician (*ruyi* 儒醫) who studied medical classics and translated medical doctrines into their own practices. The two types often overlapped: physicians with family backgrounds were likely trained in medical classics, and literati physicians were often from medical families or trained under experienced physicians.[2]

In this chapter, I use these two scholars' findings as the groundwork for understanding and interpreting modes of knowledge transmission among practitioners of traditional Chinese medicine in the Bay Area. We will explore these questions: How are the Bay Area practitioners trained? How do the schools design their curricula to satisfy the requirements of California State Acupuncture Board, and also ensure that the students are prepared for both the licensing exam and the competitive consumer market? How do these factors affect the formation of the professional identity of the practitioners in the area?

TCM SCHOOLS IN THE BAY AREA

The state of California legalizes practices of traditional Chinese medicine and the more general Oriental Medicine by licensing the practice of acupuncture. There are some TCM practitioners who forgo licensing by using noninvasive techniques such as *qigong*, cupping, and herbal supplements.[3] However, since acupuncture is the only modality in traditional Chinese medicine that is recognized and covered by health insurance providers, and since the acupuncture license legitimizes a wide range of clinical practices that may or may not actually fall under TCM's jurisdiction, most practitioners choose to acquire a state acupuncture license. In terms of starting a clinic as a business operation, which requires a business license from the city in which the clinic is located, a licensed acupuncturist is readily approved, whereas an unlicensed practitioner often faces city authorities' suspicion of possibly using the clinic (as in the case of a massage parlor with an unlicensed practitioner) for prostitution and other illegal activities.

In California, one must first graduate from an approved TCM or Oriental Medicine (OM) degree (four years/thirty-six months) or training program (three years/twenty-seven months) before taking the licensing exam. Those who had previous training in biomedical healthcare can transfer some of their past credits to shorten their TCM or OM degree programs. Seasoned practitioners from overseas can petition to use their previous training and professional experiences to satisfy this requirement, but this group of practitioners makes up a small fraction in the total practitioner pool. In other words, the majority of candidates for acupuncture license in California must complete full programs at the TCM schools.

There are six schools in the Bay Area that are approved by the California Acupuncture Board to prepare students for the state licensing exam for acupuncturists. Please see the Appendix, Figure 2, for the list of schools and their programs.

KNOWLEDGE TRANSMISSION IN THE BAY AREA TCM SCHOOLS

The class is about to start. After introducing myself to the instructor, I find a chair in the corner of the classroom. Students pour in, some with food in their hands, and others carrying books and binders, looking just like any class in any graduate program in California. They greet each other. Most pay no attention to my presence; a few nod and smile politely. They are used to visitors in the classroom, who are often touring all four accredited schools in the Bay Area to find one that is suitable.

In order to better understand the process of knowledge transmission in the schools that offer degree programs for traditional Chinese medicine in the Bay Area, I observed in three of the six local TCM schools. In two schools I was given access to all lecture and clinic classes for the period of eight weeks, with the agreement that the names of the schools would not be identified when I present my observations. In the third school I was not given access to classes, but was able to participate in an open clinic. The list of TCM schools and their programs can be found in the Appendix.

Unlike Elizabeth Hsu and Volker Scheid who studied TCM in China and enrolled into acupuncture programs officially,[4] the access I had to the local TCM programs allowed for a sampling of classes, but not participation in any one course in its entirety. However, the cross-section sampling allowed for observation in classes offered to students in different stages in their programs. I had the opportunity to observe in classes where the students had just started their first semester, and also in classes where the students were near the end of their school training. Furthermore, since one of the observed schools offers both English and Chinese degree programs, I was able to attend some of the same courses taught in each language.

The English program classes typically have twenty to twenty-five students in required courses, and anywhere from five to twenty-five students in elective courses. Chinese program classes are considerably smaller in comparison; required courses have five to ten students, and elective courses sometimes only two or three. Clinic observation and internship courses are often shared by students in English and Chinese programs, whereby the schools are able to consistently fill them to the maximum class capacities of five to twenty, depending on the level of practicum.

In terms of student demographics, the age of the students ranges from early twenties to fifties, with most them looking to be in their thirties and forties. English programs are attended mostly by Caucasian Americans, and occasionally a few Asian, Latino, and Black Americans (no more than 10 percent). Many of these students are already registered nurses, physical therapists, massage therapists, or have worked in healthcare related fields such as pharmaceuticals. There are also a few foreign MDs from Europe and South America, but they are truly a minority. The Chinese program is attended exclusively by Chinese ethnics who are fluent in the Chinese language, and the ones I encountered had no previous background in healthcare-related professions before they entered the TCM program.

CLASS FORMATS AND TEACHING STYLES

In required courses for the degree programs, the instructors are generally practitioners who are experienced and well prepared. Actual teaching styles depend mostly on the subject matter and the personalities of the instructors. The most popular format is to deliver a pre-structured lecture on general principles, and explain concepts by case studies from textbooks, other academic sources, and anecdotal examples from their own clinical practices. Technique-oriented courses would consist of some lecturing but mostly practice time where the students practice on each other. In-class student discussions are not common aside from clinical observations and counseling classes.

Most classes in both English and Chinese degree programs are structured and delivered much like courses offered in other post-secondary institutions in California.[5] Textbooks and compiled readers provide assigned readings, and instructors typically present the materials in class in the form of digested, interpreted, and restructured knowledge. The instructors filter the materials through their own experiences and understanding, and strategically provide students with points, tips, and ways to approach the subject matter or topic *du jour*. Students are generally not expected to need to read their textbooks in class, because they are busy taking notes of the personally processed knowledge now being orally and visually (through writing on the blackboard, class handouts, or a PowerPoint presentation) transmitted by their instructors. Unless the original texts or sources are central parts of the course (e.g., courses on medical classics), the emphasis is generally on the content, and not the textual presentation, of the material.

In some of the classes in the Chinese program, a few instructors choose to use another teaching format—textual commentary. In these classes, the instructors read the textbook or provide extensive quotes from classical sources (out loud and often with the texts right in front of the students), and provide definitions, explanations, interpretations, commentaries, and anecdotal examples as the readings go along. In addition, there is frequent cross-referencing to other classical and contemporary sources, often citing them in direct quotations too. In one class on Huangdi Neijing 黃帝內經, the instructor not only commented on selected original passages, she also supplemented the explanations of key terms by citing classical poems, a few idiomatic sayings (*chengyu* 成語), and referenced other well-known medical classics such as *Shanghan Lun* 傷寒論. The analysis sometimes was on the level of tracing the history of the meaning of individual Chinese characters in a given term. This level of cross-referencing is only possible when the students have general cultural and language competency to understand not only the references but also the inferences of how the network of references relate to each other. This same instructor, a young, new immigrant practitioner from China, laments that she is unable to introduce and help students in the English program (she also teaches in English) appreciate the beauty of classical Chinese medical texts.

Another instructor, an elderly practitioner from China who teaches "Introduction to TCM Principles," reads the standard textbook line by line with the students. At first I wondered why he had to recite the text, which is written in modern Chinese, to the students who can easily have understood the paragraphs by themselves. Then I noticed that he not only carefully defined and explained classical medical terminology that appeared in the text, he also commented on the presentation of the text and the specificity of the characters used and phrases constructed to define classical terminology. Furthermore, he asked the students to highlight and memorize key phrases. In other words, he took the text itself, whether in classical or modern Chinese, as seriously as the content of text. Finally, he supplemented recited sections with new scientific findings and his own clinical experiences, both in China and in the Bay Area. Different from the personally processed, re-presentation approach, this method effectively distinguished between the textbook knowledge, the voice and thoughts of the instructor, and the references that he cited.

The relationships between instructors and students are mostly warm and friendly. Regardless of ethnicities and teaching styles during class, instructors and students freely chitchat during class breaks. Sometimes students approach the instructors with not just questions related to the course itself, but also with their own health concerns. Other times instructors share their experiences operating their own clinics, or the more casual or interesting stories in their clinical encounters.

The students are generally more technology-savvy than the instructors, although some students are not much younger than the instructors. It could be that in the Bay Area, many of the students in the TCM programs had previous or even have current careers in technology-related industries. The schools are equipped with wireless internet connection, and it is common for students, especially in schools in the South Bay (where Silicon Valley is located), to take notes with their laptop computers and conduct online searches on the topic being discussed in class.

BUILDING CLINICAL EXPERIENCES

Students are immersed in the clinical experiences early on in their program. In the "Beginning Observations Theater" course, taken by students still fairly new to the program, they observe their instructor practice on volunteer patients. Each two-to-four-hour class is scheduled for seeing two to three patients, and the patients are charged a significantly lower fee compared to private sessions in the school clinic. The students are still in the process of learning rudimentary concepts and etiologies of traditional Chinese medicine, so the focus of the course is to demonstrate a standard procedure for clinic encounters and treatments. The instructor carefully demonstrates, step by step, how to greet a patient, ask the proper questions to gather enough information for diagnosis, and make the patient comfortable and informed of the treatment procedure. There are not always enough patients signed up for each class session, and students in the class routinely take turns serving as the patient, so I volunteered to be the patient for demonstration in the same course at the two different schools.

The "Beginning Observation Theater" is so standardized that it basically takes the same format in all schools. In these classes, the students are given a standardized chart that they use to document the intake, diagnosis, and treatment for each patient. The classroom has a desk for intake and a treatment table to perform acupuncture on. The instructor first greets me, and proceeds to ask detailed questions about my general physical health and subjective complaints. Then he or she checks my pulse on both wrists and describes to the class what kind of pulse is detected. My tongue is also observed, and the result is announced to the class as well. The students record that onto their own copy of the chart and are invited to come closer to look at my tongue or check my pulse if they want. After a round of basic questions by the instructor, the students are asked if they have additional questions to ask me/the patient. The instructor then proceeds to diagnose, explain the diagnosis by relating to the stated symptoms and complaints, and prescribe herbal formula (both in patent medicine and with a detailed list of herbs) appropriate for the condition. Finally the instructor announces and explains what acupuncture points should be used to treat the condition. I am invited to position myself on the treatment table, and the instructor inserts the needles into those acupuncture points announced to the class. While the needles are in, the students are encouraged to approach me to take a closer look, or to make sure that I am comfortable and warm. After about twenty-five minutes, the needles are removed by the instructor, and the class thanks me for volunteering. The students only observe at this stage, so they do not touch me except for when they want to experiment with taking pulses.

As the students advance in the degree program, they begin to observe and follow their instructors in the school clinics, where the pace is faster, and the discussions shift from establishing clinical routines to diagnoses and treatment strategies. Sometimes instructors would first let the students visit the volunteer patients, then convene them in a classroom nearby to have detailed discussions on the cases at hand, and then guide the class in designing treatment plans, which the instructor would then execute on the patients. Gradually, their clinical observations become more hands-on. Students often start to practice on patients in open clinics and ear clinics where patients have less serious conditions and are needled in mostly harmless parts of the body, like ears, arms, and legs. In one of the schools, new patients to the open clinic are required to have one private appointment for detailed intake to make sure that they do not have life-threatening conditions or conditions that require treatments beyond the common and easily accessible acupuncture points.

Finally, the students advance to internships where they practice supervised independent treatments in the appointment clinic, treating patients one-on-one. There are different levels in this category as well: from the earlier internships, where the supervisor may accompany the intern through the entire process of intake and treatment, to the most advanced internships, where the intern can independently perform the intake, make a diagnosis with the consultation of the supervisor who sits in an office nearby, and perform treatment independently. Patients are charged different rates in the school clinics depending on whether they are treated by the licensed acupuncturist instructors or the different levels of interns supervised by these instructors.

Some new graduates from the schools choose to practice in the school clinics after they first attain their licenses, partially because they want to gain more clinical experience and partially because it takes significant financial capital to start a private practice. Schools charge these new licensees overhead fees for treatments they perform in the school clinics.

COMMUNITY CLINICS

The clinic with private treatment rooms is not the only format in which the practitioners in the Bay Area offer their expertise. A second format, the community clinic, is gaining popularity in a healthcare market in dire need of low-cost preventative and general care. In a community clinic, rather than segregating the patients into individual rooms, patients all undergo treatments in one common area by a rotating team of practitioners. With the more common format of one-on-one, private-room treatments, the costs of running a clinic with space, equipment, and manpower to provide individualized services are reflected in the treatment fees. The cost range of $45 to $125 per each regular TCM treatment, herbs not included, can add up to overwhelming financial burdens for those who need long-term treatments, who do not have a health insurance plan that covers all or part of the cost, or who simply do not have the financial means to pay for medical treatments of any kind. In contrast, the community clinics are able to offer general and basic care at significantly lower fees, $5 to $10 at the school clinics and a $15-to-$40 sliding scale at the privately run community clinics.

I follow my informant Vera (see chapter 6) to the ear clinic she supervises in one TCM school. Operating with the community clinic format, where all patients are treated in one open space and by any available practitioner, the Ear Clinic practitioners and interns treat only with acupuncture points on the ears (known as auricular acupuncture). We are running a little late, and as Vera's car pulls into the school parking lot, we already see the line of waiting patients. Vera's interns have already set up the sizable classroom-turned-clinic when we walk in. Simple, plastic folding chairs line against the walls, and a folding table in the center of the room has a sign-in sheet, piles of regular patients' charts, and a plastic tub for donations (suggested donation is $5). Near the clinic entrance sits a large hot tea dispenser that fills the room with the pleasant minty fragrance of herbal tea that patients are invited to enjoy for free. Soft, calming music plays in the background. As the patients pour in, many seem to know one another, and patients chitchat while waiting and undergoing treatments.

Vera scrambles to put on her white coat (a requirement for all school clinics). In response to my amazement at the vibrancy of the clinic, she remarks:

> It is really a neighborhood's clinic, where folks in the local community come in to get treated, get better, and talk to each other. I've had people who have this idea that they should be able to meditate during their treatments, and complain that others were talking too much. I told them, this is not a place to meditate! This is a clinic! You need to find another place to do that.

Along with her two interns on duty, Vera circles the room to check in, diagnose, and treat people. People of different ethnicities and from all walks of life sit next to one another. There are twenty or so folding chairs in the room; some patients come in to get treated and leave, while others seem to settle in to socialize for the whole time. While auricular points are known to be effective for pain management, smoke cessation, and weight control, among other conditions, they are not full substitutes for whole-body acupuncture. On the other hand, it is an inexpensive way to effectively treat many health problems in the low income community.

I find a chair to sit down with the patients. On one side of me is a Hispanic grandmother who comes in for her aching knees (Vera is fluent in Spanish and converses with her); on the other side of me is a graduate student from India who takes public transit across town to come in every week to keep herself in check. In walks a young woman with a fashionable gothic outfit—black lips, black dress, black pumps—and covered in tattoos, and she sits down next to a teenage boy who is having a heated debate with the air and rocks himself back and forth.

The interns practically buzz around the room between patients like working bees. Vera sneaks by me between patients to see if I am doing all right. "Do you want a treatment?" she asks.

Even though I live in the same house as an acupuncturist, I am afraid of needles and try to avoid them as much as possible. But the feeling of *communitas* in the room, a quiet peace within the chaos of conversations, background music, and occasional yelps from pain, somehow makes me want to join in. And I like Vera. After interviewing her for almost two hours and watching her work for another hour, I have already developed trust in her and in her practice. With an unusual lack of resistance, I give in, even though I have no physical complaint that would require treatment.

Vera takes one step backward, looks at me, and leans forward again. "Graduate students are stressed and think too much. Let's do some points to help you with that."

Before I can blink three times, Vera has already stabbed my ears with three small ear needles each. Then she slides away ever so quickly. Within a minute I have dozed off into unconscious sleep, on the hard seat of a folding chair, warmly enveloped by the voices of strangers around me and a strange sense of safety.

Another TCM school offers two types of community clinics: 1) an ear clinic where patients are treated for twenty to twenty-five minutes each and with only auricular points ($5), and 2) a community clinic where the patients are treated for an average of one-and-a-half hours each, with acupuncture points on the head, the arms, and below the knees, or points that are accessible when the patients are fully clothed ($10). While both type clinics treat walk-in patients, patients of the community clinic are required to have one private session for an initial checkup and consultation. Both clinics have the same setup of furniture and take place in the same room in different allocated times.

Situated in a large classroom, this community clinic is set up with a circle of seven to ten adjustable reclining chairs that are usually used for outdoor porches. Hot herbal tea is offered, and soothing music plays in the background. Patients here don't talk to each other; the clinic supervisor and interns squat very low next to the patients, and all conversations are conducted in whispers. The lighting in the room is intentionally dimmed, and patients typically close their eyes and rest while they undergo treatment. In fact, with the unspoken consensus to keep very quiet and the light very dim, one cannot do much but rest silently or meditate. Interns retreat to one brighter corner of the room to study, when they are not busy with the patients. It seems like the perfect place for Vera's patients who are looking for a clinic where they can meditate. The supervisors sit on the side; interns do all the intakes and consult the supervisors with their findings, diagnoses, and treatment plans. With the approval of their supervisors, the interns then go and execute the treatments. The supervisors only check on the patients if the interns feel unsure or if the patients request to see them . . . or in the worst scenario, when something goes wrong.

Practitioners I have interviewed do not all talk about "community clinic" the same way. To the seasoned practitioners who emerged from the AIDS epidemics in the 1980s, a community clinic means a clinic that serves the local community and where the community forms within the clinic. It was a historically dark time for many in the gay community in San Francisco, where the mysterious yet deadly virus was wiping out a community and where the acupuncturists were often in the closest circle of those who faced death with their patients. Several practitioners who practiced in the Haight-Ashbury free clinic vividly recall both the fear and the incredible bonds that were formed between practitioners and patients, and between patients, in that fear. Vera, who is very much one of that generation of practitioners, seems to embrace that model. In the ear clinic she supervises, she not only encourages the forming of a community among the patients, she also participates in the community herself.

A newer model also called the "community clinic" has gained popularity in the Bay Area in the past three to five years. One clinic supervisor identifies the origination of this second model as the Working Class Acupuncture Clinic in Portland, Oregon. Started in 2002, the Working Class Acupuncture Clinic operates on a business model that focuses on offering affordable acupuncture to working class people. If that does not sound Marxist enough, the Working Class Acupuncture website also calls itself "the calmest revolution ever staged," with a red upraised fist as a business logo. The model has received so much attention from the acupuncture community that a Community Acupuncture Network (CAN) was formed in 2006. Without being explicitly anticapitalist, the network's stated goal is to "make acupuncture more affordable and accessible by promoting the practice of offering acupuncture in community settings for a sliding scale ranging within $15 to $40 a treatment."[6] If my experience in the second TCM school clinic is an accurate interpretation of the model, the model emphasizes making acupuncture affordable for the community (or "the People" in Marxist parlance), rather than providing a space to foster or build a community among patients.

Or perhaps it does build a community, but a community of practitioners rather than a community of practitioners and patients. There are also practitioners, like my informant Alison, who talk about a "community clinic" in which a group of practitioners not only share a business and the financial responsibilities but also form an intellectual cohort where they continue to educate one another and advance together.

The community clinics in some of the TCM schools provide students with exposure to possible alternatives to the more conventional models in the TCM profession: ones that take after biomedical clinics, or ones that take after the luxury spas. As the TCM schools continue to produce licensed acupuncturists who enter an increasingly competitive market, models that venture into serving a wider demographic not only contribute to filling the gaps in the existing healthcare system, but also create niches that satisfy the individual temperaments of practitioners and where they can better practice their craft.

CHALLENGES IN THE TCM SCHOOLS

In discussing the education provided by the TCM schools in the Bay Area, a few challenges must be brought to the foreground. From the perspective of the school administrations, they are constantly caught between different demands and interests—meeting the accreditation requirements, facing the competitive recruitment of students, finding qualified classroom instructors and clinic supervisors, and training the students to pass the state licensing exam within the three to four years. Somewhere between start and finish, the curricula should somehow provide the students enough information to become practitioners who are both clinically efficacious and theoretically competent. The TCM schools in the Bay Area each have strategies in their attempts to balance all the demands while remaining profitable as viable businesses. Among the veteran practitioners and instructors I interviewed, only one felt that the degree program alone can possibly prepare graduates adequately for independent clinical practice.

On the other hand, the student pool applying and entering the TCM schools is diverse in academic and professional backgrounds. Seasoned practitioners I have talked to have consistently found that when they were going through the TCM programs, students were predominantly older (in their thirties or older) and seeking a second career. However, current TCM school administrators and instructors are observing a shift in this trend in the past few years. The shift is not accidental: the schools have been making more recruiting efforts in college fairs, and are thus seeing more applicants who are fresh college graduates in their early twenties. Although the California State Board only requires a high school diploma for entering a training program, the Bay Area schools offer graduate level programs, and predominantly require a bachelor's degree in any field upon entering. Still, it is common to have students with little previous experience or coursework in Western sciences and healthcare in the same class with seasoned biomedical healthcare providers and body-workers. The high variation in the students' competencies in human physiology and general health-related knowledge is apparent in both English and Chinese programs, indicating that it is not a language or cultural issue. In one intermediate Chinese-language TCM "Diagnosis" class I attended, only one student out of the total of nine knew what a hernia[7] is, while the rest of the class drew a blank on the condition, not only on the English term, but also on its Chinese partial equivalent *shanqi* 疝氣[8] , which is commonly used by TCM, biomedicine, and also in Chinese folk vernacular.

In short, regardless of the language of instruction, the TCM degree programs are faced with too much material to be covered in too little time, with a wide range of "starting points" yet a relatively clearly defined "finish line." The curriculum design is further complicated by various visions of the faculty and administrators. While administrators are usually keenly aware of the reality of packing essential training into the limited time frame, faculty who are seasoned practitioners often see the necessity of providing more training in biomedical foundations. The intentions are practical. One practitioner who trains interns in her clinic explains why some biomedical training is necessary:

> When patients come in, we need to be able to determine whether we are capable of treating them. Some students don't have a sense of who is in real danger and should be sent to the ER instead. Also, how are we going to take care of our patients if we don't understand the biomedical diagnoses they get from their Western doctors, or if we don't know how to read their test results and charts?[9]

Senior practitioners (*lao zhongyi* 老中醫) from China, who had been important sources of knowledge and experiences beyond textbooks and school curricula, are leaving the schools. While some of these experienced practitioners inherited unique techniques and theories from important medical lineages, others developed their own clinical approaches over long years of practicing with large patient bases in China. These practitioners are not only underappreciated by the Bay Area TCM schools, they are also often underpaid. Jason, a practitioner who teaches and actively participates in curriculum design at one of the Bay Area schools, has tried to advance the professional image of these experienced practitioners by suggesting that his school's clinic establish the "Experts Clinic" (*zhuanjia menzhen* 專家門診). Unfortunately, the responses from the school administrators were lukewarm at best. Jason fears the possibility of actually losing these knowledge holders with passing time:

> [The school administrators don't understand that] the most important thing is to have authorities and experts teaching in the clinic. Like in my school, these senior doctors are sixty, seventy years-old, I'm the youngest among them. After these senior doctors retire, who is going to replace them? Nobody. Then [the school] just hires a few graduates from our own school who know how to teach, and run that way. I say, now I can offer my time [to run the Experts' Clinic], but [the school] needs to think about how I can be replaced eventually. I can be the front line. Now I am the expert, and the senior teachers should gather up their confidence and do the same. We have experts in gynecology, we have experts in pediatrics, and they can charge even higher than I do, I can care less.

The school administrators are not the only ones lacking enthusiasm in what Jason considers an important way of passing on clinical knowledge. The senior practitioners themselves also have reservations—many feel obligated to keep secret techniques within their own families. Jason argues against such behavior, and exclaims:

> Now, I teach anybody. We must have confidence! If every senior doctor has two to three students, and if one or two of these students end up staying in the school, they will carry on. The school must carry on. Otherwise these [senior practitioners] leave, and we don't know who is an expert anymore. Not everybody is experienced enough to be an expert, but more experts in the school is going to benefit the school.[10]

Jason also points out that the TCM schools provide almost no support for faculty who wish to conduct local clinical research. The schools' lack of funding and facilities to sponsor larger scale clinical research has implications for the cycle of knowledge transmission in the profession. These implications will be discussed later in the chapter.

THE IMPORTANCE OF CHINESE MEDICAL CLASSICS IN THE TCM EDUCATION

After more than twenty years as recognized and licensed health professionals, the TCM professionals in the Bay Area have found themselves in a competitive market that requires ever increasing sophistication in their understandings of the craft. In addition, the influx of China-trained practitioners in the recent years began to raise the question of cultural authenticity in the TCM knowledge being transmitted in the local TCM schools. Practitioners and administrators trained in China actively use their own educational experiences as references to how the school curricula can better prepare the students for clinical practices.

More coursework on, or at least more exposure to, Chinese medical classics has been an issue for the schools for many years. Advocates of more training in Chinese classics see such training as essential to both theoretical and cultural competencies of the students. As some schools transition from three-year to four-year programs, more courses that are dedicated to Chinese medical classics, such as *Huangdi Neijing*, *Jinkui Yaolüe* 金匱要略, and *Shanghan lun*, are being offered as either required courses or electives. While there are yet to be widely recognized standard English translations of the Chinese medical classics, which were written in compact and archaic classical Chinese, a few scholarly translations have emerged in the past few years as archeologically and linguistically sophisticated (for example, Unschuld's translations, and Nigel Wiseman), but not all TCM programs assign these works. Interestingly, English classes in TCM classics are usually taught by Chinese instructors who are very knowledgeable in the classics, but do not necessarily have good mastery of the English language. Not only are they often not aware of the English language literature on the classics, but also their own attempts to translate the original texts into English yield limited interpretations.

The vast majority of the students in the English language programs do not know enough Chinese to study the classics in the original. The TCM schools are gradually increasing their requirements in medical Chinese, some from one semester to two semesters. These classes attempt to cover basic medical vocabulary and possible clinic conversations. From these classes alone, students might acquire enough familiarity with a narrow range of Chinese terms to communicate with those clinic supervisors who speak limited English.

Students in the Chinese language programs are not necessarily better educated in the classics. Although these students are fluent in modern Chinese, they are not required to meet any qualification in classical Chinese. Course materials used for Chinese courses in medical classics are up to the individual instructors' discretion. Some instructors opt to use standard publications from PRC, which are sterile and filtered transliterations into modern Chinese. These textbooks cover major theoretical themes systematically, but usually give simplified and narrow interpretations. In her ethnographic work in Yunnan, China, Elizabeth Hsu also found that the government-run TCM schools often cover the medical classics only to the extent of indexing the topics and having the students memorize some of the passages.[11] Other instructors wish to retain the beauty of the classical language and teach directly from the original texts. This approach requires that the instructors themselves have the mastery over not only the classical language, but also the historical commentaries on the texts. Instructors who are California state-licensed acupuncturists (a standard bottom line when most TCM schools hire), have literary training in Chinese classics (medical and general), and have the ability to effectively articulate and teach their knowledge are rare in the Bay Area.

Unfortunately, these precious teachers are often underappreciated by the schools, their students, and even their colleagues.

For a medicine that has been rapidly growing and maturing within a foreign culture for a few decades now, TCM has reached an awkward point. For those who believe that the success of biomedicine in its savvy modernity and universality lies in its detachment from cultures, the effectiveness of TCM treatments, even as they are freely extracted from the Chinese cultural and theoretical framework, is good news. However, as some TCM practitioners and educators venture beyond merely the clinically practical, they increasingly find that, more than just language competency, cultural competency can be a crucial requirement for deeper theoretical inquiries in Chinese medicine.

Meilun, a professor who taught in medical schools in China and now teaches integrative TCM and clinical internships in Bay Area TCM schools, shares her perspective:

> Chinese medicine developed over the history of few thousand years. The development of a culture and the development of a medicine take a certain process. In that developmental process, there are always some theories that were eliminated, and other theories that are further developed. Nowadays, learning Chinese medicine in China requires learning the classics, and that is very helpful in understanding the TCM theoretical system. However, clinically, we can't only use these theories, we must combine theories with modern technology, and therefore there are two methodologies in treating illnesses [in the Chinese setting].

She outlines the limitations for non-Chinese students who study in the local TCM programs:

> For the American students, they are not able to study the theories from the four classics [in depth]. They get a very very shallow understanding of the theories, just the basics. There is no way for them to understand deeply and thoroughly. If they can't understand [these theories], their understanding for their entire system of Chinese medicine is very limited.

She feels the effect of the lack of that sense of theoretical evolution among her students in her herbal formula course. Medical theoretical schools (*yijia* 醫家) in different dynasties, she argues, are informed by the general scholarly theoretical frameworks of their respective eras. Without understanding how the general scholarly theoretical frameworks differ from dynasty to dynasty, the theoretical discrepancies between classical herbal formulae become almost impossible to reconcile. To solve this problem, she suggests a more systematic and historical analysis of TCM medical theories:

> Chinese medical history [classes] should do more than introduce what books were written in what dynasty, or what person was from what

dynasty, but go into the medical system itself. From what we see . . . *Huangdi Neijing*, a book from two thousand years ago, the Han dynasty, until today, the developments and the heritage of each dynasty. First the theory was this way, in the Sui dynasty it developed to what level, then in the Tang dynasty it developed to what level, then in the Ming dynasty it developed to what level. It is a web of [theoretical] inheritance and interconnections.

However, Meilun feels this kind of comprehension is impossible for those students in the English language program, because the existing curriculum does not include courses to foster in-depth studies of TCM theories. Furthermore, "the program is also too short, [the students] don't have the condition or the time to scrutinize this kind of stuff."[12]

Kelly, a Caucasian American practitioner who teaches and practices in integrative medicine clinics and teaches in the doctoral program in one TCM school, views the language issue in more practical terms:

> I really don't think it impacts day-to-day practice. Even less so now compared to when I went to school. We studied herbs first just by the lab names. I thought that there was going to be more of a crossover, but the only place that you could buy herbs was Chinatown.
> It's interesting because now there's a little more training around it in the schools in the language . . . when I don't think you need it as much [nowadays] because it's so easy to access products across the board. I also think that it's somewhat misleading to take a semester or two of medical Chinese at school, because it's a phenomenally difficult language to learn and I don't believe that you can really pick up that much unless what you are trying to teach is theory around the development of characters and how the importance of that is in terms of representation—that's the only way I think you would have value.

Having stated the above, Kelly also recognizes that the lack of competency in Chinese language skills may compromise the students' theoretical understanding:

> I think that [the language situation] impacts theoretical foundation. So when you're trying to emphasize the development of a new line of thinking that's based on a foundation of many different things, I think that you have a big stretch if you don't speak the original language.[13]

Alison, a Caucasian American professor who has been part of a study group that learns to translate Chinese medical classics from the Chinese original into English, tries to incorporate what she learns into her teaching:

> This term I was teaching Five Elements,[14] the two hours that I have [to cover the concept]. Instead of talking about the five elements generally and talking about just general things, I took the translation of the *Suwen* 素問. It starts out talking about the Eastern corner and wind, and all the aspects of wood, and flavor. I went through that. And I was

trying to piece by piece go through it so that people got a sense of something that is not talked about ever, which is that, when we are talking about the five elements, we are talking about the different movements of *qi*. When the *qi* manifests, we can see it in the climate, we can see it in the movements of a person, we can see it . . . it manifests in all these different forms, but there is a shared quality of that type of *qi*. That is something that, oh, no one has ever put that together, ever, in this school anyway.

Alison associates the lack of training in the classics with the Chinese Communist party's attempt to de-spiritualize the medicine by not talking about the energetic aspect of it:

It is obvious what is talked about all the time in the Five Elements school. [PRC-TCM is] the communist Chinese take on a couple thousand years of history of Chinese medicine. It leaves out a lot of the energetic nature of the medicine.

The recognition of the energetic underpinning of human health conditions is, to Alison, the core of understanding the diagnostic tools and treatment protocols in TCM. Without such recognition, the TCM can easily become merely a belief system:

If people don't get [the energetic] piece and learn TCM as just a mechanical medicine, and then just try to believe it . . . I think that is why a lot of the acupuncturists in this country don't feel confident. They don't always feel so confident in their work because they don't actually understand it. They are just trying to believe it. And that's a bad feeling.[15]

George, a Chinese herbology professor who practices and teaches what he calls "classical Chinese medicine," would say that the problem is not the lack of talking about the "energetic." He argues that non-Chinese students and practitioners are essentially incapable of understanding Chinese medicine because they do not understand the philosophical mode from which the medicine arises:

Foreigners [non-Chinese] just won't do, even if they have lived in China for many years. . . . If Americans want to understand Chinese medicine . . . I have put some thought into this, and come to no good conclusion. The impression (*xiang* 象) can only be infinitely approximated, but never quite concretely clear. This is also a characteristic of Chinese medicine. If somebody says I am completely clear about all of [these Chinese medical concepts], then that is not *zhongyi* anymore. That becomes Western medicine. For example, the Bible, this book, many people have read it for many years, but do they really understand it completely? Even the professors in the theological schools can't claim that they understand completely. Why is that? It is a classic text (*jingdian* 經典), you can try to get infinitely close, but won't ever really reach that level (*jingjie* 境界). Chinese classic texts are like that too. You can try to get infinitely close to it, but experience in the lifetime of any given person is limited.

In addition, he is of the opinion that Chinese medical theories can only be properly comprehended after extensive immersion in Chinese classics—not just the medical classics, but literary and philosophical classics—in order to understand the classical Chinese language and the particular mode of thinking:

> One needs to have substantial foundation in Chinese culture to understand Chinese medicine . . . the Four Books and Five Classics, *Daxue* 大學 and the Analects . . . [one must first have read and] understood these. Why read these things? Because Chinese medicine is one language, and Western medicine is another language. The language of Chinese medicine is completely different from that of modern science. We are conversing now using the same Chinese language (*Hanyu* 漢語), but when I speak with the specialized terms (*shuyu* 術語), it's a different language. I say we nurture *yang* in the autumn and winter, and nurture *yin* in the spring and summer. . . . If I don't explain it to you, you wouldn't know what that means. This language is different because it is a language that was developed two thousand years ago. We are people from two thousand years later . . . how are we supposed to understand the language from two thousand years ago? We can't understand. The fundamental ideas are not the same.

Whereas George sees it as nearly impossible for Chinese philosophical conceptions to transcend cultural boundaries, he argues that physical sensations are universal and should be the entry point for communication. He demonstrates his point with some cross-cultural examples:

> Things like *shanghuo* 上火 [heat rising] . . . in China, our common people (*laobaixing* 老百姓) only have to open their mouths and already talk Chinese medicine. Things like "heartache" (*xinteng* 心疼) and "You succeed in what your heart desires" (*xinxiang shicheng* 心想事成). Those are Chinese medical concepts. Shouldn't it be your head desires or your brain desires? In the West there are similar sayings. Like when you break up, your heart is broken. Why not your head is broken? Fundamentally, human feelings are shared. When a person is very sad, the head doesn't hurt, the heart hurts. When a person is only a little sad his head hurts, but when very sad, the heart hurts.
>
> The basic sensations are the same, but the Americans are not trained [in the particular vocabulary]. Communicating with the Americans takes training, and that takes the work of all acupuncturists. We need to train every patient and everyone around us. In our daily conversations we should talk about it. With constant practice, over time, they will get it. When we talk about these things repeatedly they will get it.[16]

RECAP: LANGUAGE AND CULTURAL COMPETENCY AS THE KEY TO ACCESS KNOWLEDGE

The TCM schools in the Bay Area recruit students from all walks of life; among the admitted students, some had very little or no background in Western sciences or healthcare, and those who enter the English programs mostly have no background in Chinese language or culture. The school curricula aim to train all students to become competent clinicians by the end of the masters level program, and in response to popular demand for more exposure to the Chinese medical classics, have increased course requirements for Chinese medical terms and medical classics within the limited scheduling space within the compact programs. Chinese ethnic instructors, who are undoubtedly strong and authoritative knowledge brokers in the TCM schools, express the difficulty (or impossibility) for non-Chinese ethnic students to fully understand TCM, which, to the China-trained instructors, is embedded in and informed by the Chinese language and culture, theoretically and clinically. As torch holders and gatekeepers, Chinese ethnic instructors insist that real and substantial TCM knowledge can only be accessed by those who are linguistically and culturally competent. The access is not necessarily determined by ethnicity—as Rafael will share in chapter 8. Although he was not ethnically Chinese, the fact that he spoke fluent Mandarin Chinese prompted his Chinese instructor to grant him access to discussions in *Yijing* 易經 and Chinese cosmology.

Furthermore, the goal of limited access seems to be more than just to keep knowledge inside a small circle; instead, as George suggests, those who come to the medicine should be educated to adjust to it, rather than the medicine adjusting to those who do not have full understanding of the larger cosmological context. Authenticity becomes a powerful capital here, where the Chinese cultural interpretations are held in high esteem.

Instructors who are not Chinese ethnics, especially those who do not possess high Chinese language and cultural competency, focus on the practicality of TCM. Recognizing that not understanding the Chinese language and culture can be a shortcoming in understanding TCM, they point out the importance of the energetic aspect of TCM. Beyond words, the energetic or *qi* can be experienced universally after some training. Furthermore, it is the acupuncture, the needling, that treats health conditions, and the healing transcends cultural interpretations of the medical theories.

It is interesting that these two positions on access to TCM knowledge each grants instructors with some power, but different powers are granted in each position. Cultural and linguistic specificity secures the status of authenticity and resists accommodation to the American mainstream, and universality offers the exact opposite, which is the liberty to accommodate to the needs of the patients based on the subjective experiences of the practitioners and patients in the clinical setting.

STATE REQUIREMENTS, SCHOOL CURRICULA, AND IDENTITY FORMATION

The California State Acupuncture Board sets the basic curricular standards for educational institutions that train and prepare students for the licensing exam. Although the TCM schools in the Bay Area offer programs that grant masters degrees to prepare for licensure and doctoral degrees for post-licensure, the State Acupuncture Board states only two years of baccalaureate level education as entrance requirement.[17] Rather than naming the level of degree program and allowing for individual school variations, the State Board requires that the training program consists of at least 1,548 hours of theoretical training, 800 hours of clinical training, and that "the coursework shall extend over a minimum period of four academic years, eight semesters, twelve quarters, nine trimesters, or thirty-six months."[18] Depending on the individual needs and preferences of the students, the Bay Area schools offer different "tracks" that allow students to complete the programs in three to four years, very often while also working full-time jobs. In order to finish in three years, the students would have to continuously attend school full-time every semester/quarter/trimester, with no summer breaks.

The Bay Area schools clearly identify themselves as graduate-level institutions, and recruit students at college job fairs rather than targeting new high school graduates. Students who enter these programs usually have at least an associate degree, and many have bachelor's degrees and above.[19] The State Board attempts to compensate for this wide variation in educational backgrounds among entrants by requiring 400 hours of coursework in (Western) general sciences that can be satisfied with transferred units if the students have completed them elsewhere as part of their bachelor's degree programs. Perhaps also to better qualify the programs for granting graduate level degrees, the schools also uniformly require significantly more hours of both theoretical and clinical training than mandated by the State Board.

While the Board's definition of clinical training is straightforward, its outline of theoretical training provides room for interpretation that results in each school building their curricula in support of several different models for traditional Chinese medicine. Below is a brief overview of the state requirements for theoretical training that prepares for acupuncture licensure:[20]

General Sciences (400 hours)

- General biology, chemistry, physics, anatomy, and physiology.
- General psychology, including counseling skills

- Pathology
- Nutrition and vitamins

History of medicine and medical terminology (30 hours)

- History of medicine: "survey of medical history, including transcultural healing practices"
- Medical terminology

Clinical medicine, other healthcare practices, and first aid (128 hours)

- Clinical sciences: "a review of internal medicine, pharmacology, neurology, surgery, obstetrics/gynecology, urology, radiology, nutrition and public health"
- Clinical medicine: "a survey of the clinical practice of medicine, osteopathy, dentistry, psychology, nursing, chiropractic, podiatry, and homeopathy to familiarize practitioners with the practices of other health care practitioners"
- Western pharmacology
- First-aid and CPR (8 hours)

Oriental Medicine theories, acupuncture, acupressure, and breathing techniques (660 hours)

- Traditional Oriental Medicine
- Acupuncture anatomy and physiology
- Acupuncture techniques: needling, moxabustion, and electroacupuncture
- Acupressure (*tuina* or *shiatsu*)
- Breathing techniques: *Qigong*
- Traditional Oriental exercise: *Tai Chi Chuan*

Oriental Herbology (300 hours)

- Traditional Oriental herbology including botany

Practice Management and Ethics (30 hours)

- Practice management
- Ethics relating to the practice of acupuncture

It is interesting that the language used by the State Acupuncture Board is unspecific about what "medicine" entails or indicates. Under clinical medicine, the Board lists "the clinical practice of medicine, osteopathy, dentistry, psychology, nursing, chiropractic, podiatry, and homeopathy,"[21] a list that suggests a biomedical framework with recognized specialties and modalities, where "medicine" obviously equates with Western biomedicine. On the other hand, the description for medical history as "survey of medical history, including transcultural healing practices" opens up wide space for how "medicine" can be interpreted.

By interpreting these requirements, the Bay Area TCM schools offer curricula along the spectrum between three models (my categorizations): East-West Dichotomy, Integration with Biomedicine, and Pluralistic Coexistence.

In the first model, the curricula are designed to contrast between East and West, where traditional Chinese medicine represents the East and biomedicine represents the West. The language used, whether in the course titles and descriptions or in some of the instructors' and administrators' verbal expressions, emphasizes the differences between East and West. Curricula that are designed with this first model offer courses that are either East or West with little connections made between systems. ACCHS (Academy of Chinese Culture and Health Sciences) in Oakland and UEWM (University of East West Medicine) in Sunnyvale, both of which offer degree programs in Chinese and English, adhere mostly to this model. Courses that do not fall under traditional Chinese medicine are specified by West, such as Western medical modalities, Western Pharmacology, and so on. Other times the "West" is implied, such as "medicine," which defaults as biomedicine.

In the second model, there is an emphasis on integrating traditional Chinese medicine into biomedicine, with varying degrees of integration—from integrating traditional Chinese medical practices into biomedical settings to fully integrating medical theories and paradigms. This model acknowledges the dominance of the biomedical paradigm, but also actively promotes the incorporation of more traditional Chinese medical strategies into biomedical treatment plans. ACTCM (American College of Traditional Chinese Medicine) in San Francisco and AIMC (Acupuncture & Integrative Medicine College) in Berkeley offer curricula that are strongly supportive of this model. ACTCM has a long history of relationships with local biomedical hospitals and centers where their students can experience more integrative practices. Many graduates from ACTCM continued to foster this model by working closely or as part of biomedical institutions.

Lastly, the third model recognizes what the other two models pay little attention to: there are many other healing practices and paradigms besides biomedicine and traditional Chinese medicine that also coexist in the shared sociocultural space. Practitioners find it helpful to establish understandings and working relationships with other alternative medical systems and modalities, because often the patients undergo several alternative therapies simultaneously. Understanding other healing practices not only allows practitioners to serve their patients better, it also provides practitioners with deeper understandings of possible competitors with a similar client base. FBU (Five Branches University) in San Jose shows consideration in this direction by including in its required one-unit Medical Modalities course guest speakers who may be a "general practitioner (MD), surgeon, pharmacist, chiropractor, neurologist, podiatrist, osteopath, gynecologist, oncologist, public healthcare nurse, homeopath, naturopath, shaman, and ayurvedic practitioner."[22] There has always been a small group of licensed TCM practitioners in the Bay Area who incorporate other alternative medical modalities and healing philosophies into their practices of traditional Chinese medicine. Other practitioners may not incorporate other systems into their own practice, but learn through their patients about other healing practices and sometimes even work closely with other healers.

It is important to recognize that all programs aim to train their students to first and foremost become practitioners of TCM, so the differences between the models are subtle and mostly ideological rather than technical. In other words, the graduates from these programs would all have the training in performing proper acupuncture and herbal medicine, but how they conceptualize traditional Chinese medicine within the Californian context and the biomedical framework can be largely shaped by the particular curricula that they were trained in. Indeed, when I interviewed practitioners in the Bay Area, they also conceptualized traditional Chinese medicine in a range between these three models. Many of my informants were also educators, administrators, and instructors in the schools, where they further reinforced these models by designing the curricula and courses with their conceptualization of traditional Chinese medicine within the Californian context. As a result, a range of professional identities for practitioners are formed and reinforced as the cycle of knowledge transmission continues.

The list of Bay Area TCM schools and programs can be found in the Appendix, Figure 2.

IDENTITY FORMATION IN CLASSROOM IMAGINATION

As discussed previously, there seems to be a loosely shared ideological conception among the practitioners in the Bay Area of not only the clinical practices, but also the appearance and atmosphere in the clinical space. When I audited in the TCM schools, I was pleasantly surprised to find that what I previously observed as shared yet largely unarticulated ideals are concretely and explicitly discussed in the classrooms. In other words, the practitioners who run private practices not only decorate their clinics in a fashion that they collectively feel would appeal to their intended clientele, but also their ideals are now becoming codified knowledge and part of formal coursework.

While not all TCM schools in the Bay Area emphasize the business aspect of clinical practice equally, it is increasingly recognized that some training in marketing and business planning greatly increases the success rate of their graduates. After all, even among the informants in this study, who make up only a small percentage of the licensed and unlicensed practitioners in the Bay Area, there are already examples of clinically skillful and experienced practitioners who suffer financially and emotionally because of their lack of training in operating a business.

In one school in which I observed, students are required to complete a series of four courses totaling only four units. Since students are less burdened by coursework, clinic internships, and preparation for the licensing exam in the earlier phases of their programs, many students attend these courses when they still have little technical knowledge and few clinical skills. On the other hand, giving students the opportunity to imagine their careers early on in the program probably also helps them decide their professional directions. Do they want to open their own private practices? Or join an established practice? Or join with a few fellow practitioners and start a community clinic? Or perhaps stay and teach at the school?

The "Practice Building" series mostly focuses on the minutia of starting a solo clinic, which is still by far the most commonly preferred form of practice arrangement, perhaps followed by the joint practice that saves on rent, shares equipment, and often provides the important professional and personal companionship that some practitioners value highly. It is interesting that because the profession does not require the residency or apprenticeship phase where practitioners can gradually evolve from being a student into a fee-charging professional, a large part of the Practice Building training is to help students present themselves as experienced professionals as soon as they open the clinic door for business. Precisely because the newly minted practitioners are not very experienced, all other details of the practice, from clinic decoration, movement flow in the clinic space, the actual treatment routine, and the fee-charging procedure must all be carefully considered and planned to compensate for the lack of clinical experience. Granted, even for experienced practitioners, a clinic that appeals to or even attracts clients can greatly enhance their market competitiveness.

In the Practice Building class I attended, the students were working on their semester-long project: a marketing or business plan for their imaginary practice. The students were asked to consider as minutely as possible all aspects of their practices and to articulate and outline their individual purpose and mission and their analysis of their starting points, conduct market research on their potential competitors and on setting appropriate fees, and construct strategies to promote themselves by emphasizing their strengths and packaging their weaknesses. Grid diagrams and marketing models were presented to the students as a basis for their project.

Another class on practice management led the students through the planning of setting up the clinic so that it would be ready for business. The students were asked to brainstorm exactly how they would or should set up the clinic, room by room, furniture by furniture, item by item. The instructor, Paul, quickly wrote down items on the whiteboard, and affirmed the students' enthusiastic ideas. A collective excitement formed through the process of what seemed like a verbal/visual concretization of ideals, if not fantasies, which were "grounded" by the confirmations or at least commentaries of the instructor.

"When the first client walks in, the clinic should look clean, but seem like it's been working for a few years," Paul suggested. "The good thing about us is that most people don't know much about acupuncture, so they don't have lots of expectations of how we run the practice," he further articulates.

So succinctly, Paul pointed to the key aspects of how some practitioners succeed in running a business with the medicine. First, even if actual clinical experiences are lacking, a comfortable and lived-in atmosphere helps provide a sense of grounding and even professional credibility. Also, an awareness of the relative plasticity and malleability of TCM as an alternative medicine is the starting point for creative incorporations and manipulations of resources. I could not help but think about the few practitioners I know personally who could benefit from these considerations, but at the same time wondered if it would have been their worst nightmare if they were required to think about anything related to business at all. Alternatively, the systematization of a market-driven business model for the profession is exactly what some practitioners chose this form of medicine in order to avoid. It seems that the domination of the profit-driven market machine is utterly inescapable.

Spunky and youthfully energetic, Paul designed and taught the Practice Building series I observed. A Caucasian American in his early thirties, he exuded the corporate attitude with upbeat, affirmative language and marketing parlance. Although only a recent graduate from the school he works in and with only one year as a licensed acupuncturist, his previous experiences as a founder of a martial arts group, a teacher in peaceful resolutions to conflicts, and a consultant for non-profit organizations qualified him for a multi-tasking job in the school. He is in charge of admissions and internet technology support, and he teaches as well. On top of so many different roles to play in the school, Paul has a small private practice in Sacramento, California, where he rents one room in a clinic to see patients two days a week.[23]

Paul is clearly on the administrator's track that many in the profession resist or find difficult to balance. Adam, a former school administrator (see chapter 6), shares that the burden of administrative duties and the requirement of abundant and continuously cultivated clinical experiences in TCM school administrators made it challenging for the schools to find individuals who are both willing and qualified. Incidentally, in both of the schools where I observed, there were young (in their early thirties) administrators who were clinical rookies, but brought with them corporate working experience. The schools seemed to be cultivating them in ongoing clinical practices, teaching experiences, and administrative responsibilities. Most significantly, the "new blood" design and create new and market-competitive programs for the schools. Aware of the changing demographics of the students entering TCM programs (shifting from midlife, second-career students to new college graduates), the schools are clearly attentive to the need for administrators who understand this new, younger generation of prospective students and TCM trainees.

In another school, Ming, a Chinese American woman, also in her early thirties, finds herself running the Chinese language master's program, attending the Chinese language doctoral program that is in the process of seeking accreditation (the school's own administrators make up the first class of the program for the purpose of accreditation), and actively participating in the design and coordination of the doctoral program. Having previously worked in the high tech industry and the mother of two young children, Ming was immediately hired for the administrative position upon her graduation from the masters program in another TCM school in the area. In short, she has minimal clinical experience as a practitioner. On the other hand, her fluency in both English and Chinese and the confidence and assertiveness that she evinces, courtesy of her work experiences as an engineer in the Silicon Valley, prove to be essential assets for her administrative roles.[24]

There is also an attempt to address the dilemma of having either Chinese professors who have "authentic knowledge" but inadequate English skills to articulate their wisdom to non-Chinese students, or Caucasian American professors who are excellent presenters and teachers but have insufficient Chinese skills to access knowledge produced in Chinese. Wei, a young Chinese immigrant who looks like she is in her late twenties or early thirties, teaches with incredible mastery of classical Chinese texts (medical and otherwise) and extremely fluent English although even she laments the loss of beauty of the classical texts after translation. Wei has a background in teaching American and European students who study TCM in China. Her training and experiences in cross-cultural teaching, specifically in teaching the medicine, bridges the gap between those students who lack Chinese language and cultural competency and the bulk of TCM knowledge that was previously inaccessible to the majority of non-Chinese students.[25]

Wei is a full-time faculty member and administrator at the school, and practices in the school clinic. It is quite obvious why the school would be cultivating her: she is equipped to help advance the level and depth of classroom teaching. Most Chinese immigrant practitioners who have to learn English from scratch take at least seven to ten years to be able to teach coherently in English, and very often they never reach the level of fluency that does their own medical knowledge justice in the classroom. In contrast, Wei, who has only been in the United States for a little more than a year, is still very close to the pulse of the TCM knowledge-producing sources in China, and has access to the newest findings and technological advancements. As a bonus, she is an extraordinarily gifted teacher who infuses her classroom teaching with lively anecdotes and real passion for the knowledge she transmits. Best yet, she is technologically savvy, which is helpful in linking TCM teaching with the needs of a student body that is increasingly reliant on technological learning aids and sources such as power point presentations, e-mail communications, and online databases and search engines. In brief, she embodies the best of both worlds in terms of teaching TCM in an English-speaking classroom.

APPRENTICESHIPS IN PRIVATE CLINICS

Before there were TCM schools and degree programs, TCM students learned their trade from correspondence programs and old-fashioned clinic apprenticeship. These students worked for no pay or very little pay in an herb dispensary and/or clinic, and learned how to become a practitioner through long years of observing how their teachers practiced. For much of the history of medicine in China, this was the most prominent method of knowledge transmission.

As described previously, to be eligible to take the acupuncture license exam in California, whether through one of the TCM degree programs or other training programs, one must have at least 800 hours of clinical instruction.[26] As part of the degree program, these clinical hours are satisfied by hands-on clinical practice with gradually decreasing levels of supervision. There is no required "residency" after a student completes the degree program and passes the licensing exam.

It is a shared understanding that, aside from those already experienced practitioners from overseas, few new licensees are truly ready to practice independently. Some new licensees join the practices of seasoned practitioners, where they gain more experience and confidence and—it is hoped—a steady client base. Both the California Acupuncture Board and the National Certification Commission for Acupuncture and Oriental Medicine (NCCAOM) encourage seasoned practitioners to take on interns by allowing clinical teaching hours to be used as part of required continuing education credit for license renewal.

Some established TCM practitioners also take on new licensees to train in their expanding networks of clinics. One such practitioner I interviewed, who also teaches in one of the TCM schools, plans on opening three more practices in the next few years. He hires new licensees, who were his own students in the school, to be trained and mentored under his wings. When they are ready to practice independently, he will staff them in the new practices. Ultimately he aims to have his students provide the healthcare while he gradually focuses more fully on clinic administration and teaching.[27]

Su Daifu, the *zhenggu* (musculoskeletal adjustment) specialist (see chapter 4), takes interns from the local TCM schools. As Scheid observes in his fieldwork in China, that there are different types of master/apprentice relationships among practitioners of Chinese medicine, which I also observe in Su Daifu's clinic. Su Daifu has six to seven interns rotating in his clinic. All of them are there to observe his treatments and receive impromptu mini-lectures on the techniques. The students are charged a fee for each day they are present in his clinic just as they would be to intern in any private or school-run clinic. In general, Su Daifu pays little attention to which students come in and out, but during meal hours he always makes sure that the students have some money (he would often reach into his pockets and hand them whatever wrinkled up cash he finds) to buy food from nearby eateries.

One of the students, let us call him Sam, has interned with Su Daifu for longer than the rest, and has over time developed a much closer relationship with Su Daifu. Sam is a Caucasian American, but has learned to speak some Chinese from his Taiwanese girlfriend. Of all the interns, Su Daifu refers only to Sam as his *tudi*, or apprentice, while referring to the other interns as *xuesheng*, or students. As with the traditional *shi-tu* 師徒; (master-disciple) relationship, the relationship is deeper and expected to last for a lifetime, much like a father-son relationship. There is a popular Chinese idiom, "Master for one day, father for life (*yiri weishi, zhongsheng weifu* 一日為師，終生為父)," that describes the depth and commitment of such relationships. Unlike the other interns, who only observe, Sam also helps with general cleaning of the clinic and paperwork for health insurance companies. When too many patients crowd the waiting room, Sam is the only one asked to start the basic muscle relaxation part of the treatments in available rooms. Su Daifu not only gives Sam more responsibilities in the clinic, he also provides Sam with assistance, even if the help is not clinic or training related. For a short period when Sam could not afford to pay rent and was without a place to stay, Su Daifu let him sleep on the couch in the clinic office at night.

Su Daifu complains about the other interns who frequent his clinic, especially those who do not show proper respect:

> They come whenever they want, and leave whenever they want. There are days when Sam has classes and my clinic needs help, but none of the students show up. And they don't even call to tell me ahead of time. Sometimes they come in and don't bother to even say hi to me.

The interns, who are mostly Caucasian American and Chinese American, attend an English program in the nearby TCM school and speak and understand very little, if any, Chinese. Su Daifu, on the other hand, speaks almost no English. The interns often observe without really knowing what Su Daifu is saying to them. During a few of my observations, Su Daifu conveniently made me translate for his interns; the interns uniformly showed great relief and frantically wrote in their notebooks. Perhaps visual observation alone can provide the students some insight into the manual techniques, but the mini-lectures I translated for Su Daifu described the different styles of *zhenggu* and *tuina* in China, and the central strategies used in each of the styles cannot be taught without clear and precise verbal communication.

Su Daifu wants to record his knowledge, but after long work hours at the clinic each day, he finds neither time nor energy to write. At times he hinted at making me his *gan nu-er* 乾女兒 (sort of an adopted daughter) so that he could pass on his knowledge for me to write down. It is interesting that he never suggested that I become his second *tudi*, because he knew I have neither the professional training nor the technical skills to become a clinical apprentice. On the other hand, it would be appropriate for him to pass on secret knowledge to me if I were his adopted daughter, which would keep secrets "in the family."

Am I going to take up the offer to access the "secret knowledge," the reader might ask? As much as I respect Su Daifu as a practitioner and adore him as a friend, I do not intend to adopt another father, which in the Confucian system would mean lifelong filial piety, or at least the commitment to care for and respect him as I would the elders in my own family.

INTERNSHIPS IN CHINA

Some practitioners gain clinical experiences through internships in TCM hospitals and/or clinics in China. Many major TCM hospitals in China offer internships for foreigners (often taught by local doctors who speak fluent English), including Chinese practitioners from abroad. Compared to TCM clinics in the Bay Area, whether of the schools or private, TCM hospitals in China are monumentally larger in scale, patient base, and the variety of ailments they treat. Whereas a TCM school clinic might see ten to fifteen patients in one afternoon, a clinic in a TCM hospital in China routinely sees 100 to 200 patients in the same time frame, treating them with amazing speed and accuracy. Furthermore, TCM doctors in China have the authority to incorporate biomedical strategies and treatments into their practice, and also new experimental and invasive treatments based on TCM theories. American students are unable to utilize many of these "out-of-bounds" practices at home, but experiences such as these provide interns with deeper understandings of and appreciation for integrative medicine.

Besides rapid exposure to massive numbers of patients, internship in China seems to grant Bay Area practitioners an additional aura of authenticity in their practices, whatever their ethnicity may be. It is a routine practice for Bay Area practitioners who have interned in China (even just for a few months) to prominently feature the experience on their personal biographies, advertisements, and clinic websites.

NOTES

1. Hsu, *The Transmission of Chinese Medicine*, 2.
2. Scheid, *Chinese Medicine in Contemporary China: Plurality and Synthesis*, 169.
3. No license is required for herbalists.
4. See Hsu, *The Transmission of Chinese Medicine* and Scheid, *Chinese Medicine in Contemporary China: Plurality and Synthesis*.
5. This comparison is based on the author's personal experiences attending postsecondary institutions in California (University of California, Davis; Graduate Theological Union, Berkeley; University of California, Berkeley; and College of San Mateo).
6. See Community Acupuncture Network website, http://www.communityacupuncturenetwork.org/ (accessed August 17, 2009).
7. Hernia is a condition where part of an inner organ falls through a weakened abdominal wall; or it sometimes refers to spinal content protruding through the gaps between spinal columns.
8. *Shanqi* 疝氣 usually refers to herniation of intestines.
9. Personal communication, April 26, 2008.
10. Personal interview, April 24, 2008. The interview was conducted in Mandarin Chinese.
11. Hsu, *The Transmission of Chinese Medicine*, 159.
12. Personal interview, October 18, 2008. The interview was conducted in Mandarin Chinese.
13. Personal interview, August 12, 2008. The interview was conducted in English.
14. This is a common alternative to the term "Five Phases."
15. Personal interview, November 12, 2008. The interview was conducted in English.
16. Personal interview, October 18, 2008. The interview was conducted in Mandarin Chinese.
17. See Stephen Prothero, *American Jesus: How the Son of God Became a National Icon* (New York: Farrar, Straus and Giroux, 2003).
18. Ibid.
19. According to the 2006 survey I administered, outside of their TCM training, 33 percent of the practitioner informants had bachelor level degrees and 41 percent had graduate level degrees (MA, MS, PhD, and/or MD). Only 6 percent had only associate degrees before entering the TCM programs.
20. See Prothero, *American Jesus: How the Son of God Became a National Icon*.
21. Ibid.
22. See Five Branches University webpage on course descriptions, http://www.fivebranches.edu/masters-in-tcm/master-programs/527 (accessed July 5, 2009).
23. Personal interview, October 8, 2008. The interview was conducted in English.
24. Personal interview, October 13, 2008. The interview was conducted in English.
25. Personal interview and observation, October 22, 2008. The interview was conducted in Chinese, and the classes I observed in were also instructed in Chinese.
26. See California Acupuncture Board website: http://www.acupuncture.ca.gov/pubs_forms/laws_regs/art35.shtml#1399436 (accessed July 6, 2009).
27. Personal communication, April 24, 2008.

FOUR
TCM Healers in the Chinese Community

Historically, Chinese medicine has been pluralistic not just in medical theories but also in practical modalities. The craft of healing injuries and diseases has always been performed by a number of different types of healers. There are of course practitioners who primarily use acupuncture. Besides acupuncturists, three major types of TCM practitioners can be found in the Chinese ethnic community in the Bay Area: herbalists, manual healers, and ritual healers. Individual healers may incorporate more than one modality into their practices. Healers who use one of these non-acupuncture modalities also are and should be considered practitioners of traditional Chinese medicine, as they contribute to the Chinese conceptions of the medical professionals.

Although acupuncture is the only TCM modality that requires a license to practice in California, the legal definition of the scope of practice of a licensed acupuncturist includes many other modalities: "oriental massage, acupressure, breathing techniques, exercise, heat, cold, magnets, nutrition, diet, herbs, plant, animal, and mineral products, and dietary supplements to promote, maintain, and restore health" (B&P 4937 [a]-[b]),[1] as well as cupping and moxibustion (B&P § 4927 [d]).[2] Most of these non-acupuncture modalities do not involve invasive procedures (whereas acupuncture involves the insertion of needles into the patients), and are in fact practiced commonly in Chinese ethnic households and by non-licensed healers.

The Chinese ethnic community commonly equates the state acupuncture license as a license for traditional Chinese medicine in general. Therefore, some practitioners, even though they may not use acupuncture as the main modality of their healing practices, still go through TCM schools and obtain the state acupuncture license to legitimize their practices. Furthermore, being licensed as acupuncturists allows them to make health insurance claims for their treatments, and also provides the protection of malpractice insurance.

LINDA: THIRD-GENERATION ACUPUNCTURIST[3]

Linda comes from a family of TCM practitioners trained and practice in Mainland China. Her grandfather, who passed away before the family immigrated to the United States, was a very famous doctor in Guangzhou, known for his legendary skills in pulse diagnosis and TCM treatments. Her father (ear, nose, and throat specialist), uncle (father's brother; internal medicine), and aunt (uncle's wife; gynecologist) were trained in the integrated biomedicine-TCM system in the state medical schools in China. Without American biomedical credentials, Linda's father, uncle, and aunt have practiced TCM in San Francisco's Chinatown for almost forty years. They are well-known not only as TCM practitioners, but also as leaders (especially her aunt) in the TCM community for their active participation in legalization of TCM and in attaining better working conditions for the TCM practitioners in California.

The elders in Linda's family represent an important era of transformation in the medical system in Mainland China. Sponsored by the state, TCM as a tradition of healing was reformed to incorporate the biomedical paradigm—the physical-oriented anatomy, disease classifications and diagnoses, and most importantly, administration of modern pharmaceutical products. This PRC-TCM[4] system allows doctors, who are trained and given the authority over modalities in biomedicine and TCM, to utilize the most effective approaches under a wide range of possible circumstances. When PRC-TCM doctors immigrate to the United States, very few of them have the resources to meet the requirements for biomedical credentials here—to graduate from U.S. accredited medical schools, pass medical board exams, and complete residency in American biomedical hospitals, all of which require not only tremendous financial means, but also high fluency in English. More often the PRC-TCM practitioners acquire the acupuncture license, and limit their clinical practices to only using modalities that are legally allowed under the acupuncture scope of practice. Some of these practitioners teach courses on Western medicine in the local Chinese-language TCM programs, even though they do not practice biomedicine in the United States.

Still a child when her family immigrated to the United States, Linda was raised and educated in the Bay Area. Her parents only wanted the best for her. After she graduated from UC, Berkeley, with a degree in molecular cell biology, she was encouraged to apply for biomedical schools. It was obvious why the family did not immediately suggest that Linda carry on the family torch. Biomedical doctors are much more respected both in the American and the Chinese societies, and they make much more money than the TCM practitioners. Linda's father was respected in Chinatown and always had a busy practice, but he was making only a fraction of what a biomedical family physician would make. He saw many more patients than younger, less experienced practitioners, but often at a much lower rate as well. The demographics of Chinatown include a large number of elders who are covered by MediCal, which pays Linda's father $15 per treatment. The current market rate for acupuncture outside of Chinatown is $60 to $120 per session.

Linda's father never could afford to hire an assistant, so Linda has helped with the insurance claims paperwork since she was very young. Every week or two he would bring home a thick stack of charts, and Linda would type up claims to the insurance companies on a typewriter. When she was finally done with one stack, he would bring home another stack. There were always more in the clinic. It was not until recently that Linda, who is now married, has a school-age son, and is working two jobs, taught her father to fill out insurance forms by hand.

When Linda graduated from college, she did not feel that biomedicine was her calling. She started a career as a microbiology analyst in a pharmaceutical company, and found her job both fascinating and rewarding. Her parents were always supportive of her career choice, and she continued to work as the free family support for insurance processing. When a tumor on her back considerably compromised her physical health, her father gently suggested that she attend some classes in the local TCM schools to "learn how to take care of yourself." Very soon she found herself excelling through the entire program, whereupon her father hinted that she "might as well go for the licensing exam."

"Yeah, he tricked me into [TCM]," Linda says half-jokingly. "He was so happy too. He was like, yes yes! Then I got my license, and he was like yes yes yes! I said, you know, I have to open up my own business."

Rather than starting her solo practice in the very competitive Chinese market that includes her own family, Linda chose to open her own practice in a town that is very far from Chinatown. Her clinic is located in a relatively newly developed area in the Bay Area with a very small Chinese population, and few acupuncturists. She understands that starting her practice in such an area presents a different set of challenges—the most important one being that she has a local demographic that knows very little about TCM and has little previous exposure to acupuncture. On the other hand, instead of plunging directly into it as a full-time career, she kept her pharmaceutical job, where she works sixty hours each week, and only sees patients on Saturdays. Also, in this new town, where the average real estate value is much lower than that of the core regions in the Bay Area, she was able to purchase her clinic space rather than having to lease it. Ownership of the clinic space gives Linda further flexibility in building her practice part-time without the burden of monthly leasing expenses and the inevitable inflation in lease payments in the future.

I ask her if her family's legacy is a burden, and she responds with a treasured family story. Her grandfather was known for being able to accurately detect pregnancy through only pulse diagnosis—not only was he able to know if a woman is pregnant within a month of conception, he could also identify the gender of the fetus. Unfortunately, the skill was lost with the demise of her grandfather, before the family even left China. However, the skill left the family with a gift:

> I know my brother was probably saved by [the pulse reading]. It was 1970, and they hadn't implemented the one child policy yet. My mom was pregnant with [her second child], and life was hard, so she was thinking, should I abort the child or not? My grandfather felt her pulse and said, no, you shouldn't abort this one, because this is a boy. So she kept him and it was a boy, and I have a brother.

Linda has interned with her father, uncle, and aunt. Their long years of practice, both in major hospitals in China and in San Francisco's Chinatown, have granted them experiences that served as invaluable lessons to Linda. Now that she has her own practice, she still consults with them when she encounters challenging cases:

> [The elders] have been very patient with me. Anytime I have a question they are always there to answer my question. I don't think they are especially happy when I ask [laughs], but I could tell that no matter how busy they are, they always drop what they are doing to listen to what I have to say.

The elders are also Linda's role models for becoming a better TCM practitioner:

> I like working with them. They tell me, when you see a patient, you have to be very open and honest with them. Also you need to know what you need to say, you have to present yourself in a certain way, the type of training that you won't get from anywhere else.

GU DAIFU: HERBALIST[5]

Although acupuncture has been used in the Chinese societies for at least two thousand years, it was never a dominant modality. During the Ming dynasty (1368–1644), a revival in acupuncture made it more popular than before, but herbal prescriptions were always the most utilized strategy for both healing and general maintenance of health. Medicine shops usually have a resident *daifu* 大夫 (doctor) to diagnose and prescribe appropriate formulae to their clients. Independent *daifu* may also provide their services at a small stand on the street, in a tea house, from the *daifu*'s own house, or by making home visits. Before the image of the Western biomedical doctors became the standard for medical doctors, herbal *daifu* were the elite healers who occupied the center stage of the medical scene. They generated the prominent medical theories and transmitted their clinical experiences through records of their case studies. Today, herbal medicine is still the most prominent branch in traditional Chinese medicine in Chinese societies. Although acupuncture has become the most widely utilized modality of traditional Chinese medicine in the United States, herbal remedies still remain the defining modality of Chinese medicine for Chinese ethnic communities.

Gu Daifu has practiced in San Francisco's Chinatown for about fifteen years. Coming from a family lineage of herbal healers, he spent his entire life steeped in daily practices in his family's herb shop in Hangzhou 杭州, located by the famed Xihu 西湖, a beautiful lake frequented by poets and literati throughout Chinese history. He was also trained by a state-run medical school to specialize in Chinese herbal medicine.

Life in Chinatown is noisy and crowded, but Gu Daifu finds comfort in the fact that he doesn't have to speak English at all. Better yet, he can conveniently purchase the freshest produce, live chickens, and fish butchered right at the counter, and best quality herbs and patent medicines imported from China. Although he doesn't speak the Taishan 台山 dialect that is most commonly spoken in the local Cantonese community, Chinatown is still the best of both worlds that he tries to live in simultaneously—a place where he can live almost as he would in China while his only son can be educated in America. Mrs. Gu works in one of the shops down the street from where they live, which does not require that she speak any English at all.

Gu Daifu opened an herbal practice almost immediately after he set foot in America. His older brother, who came a few years before he did and also practices herbal medicine, already had an established practice in Chinatown. They knew that there was still growing demand in the community for experienced herbal doctors like them. At first, Gu Daifu used one side of the living room in the small apartment he and his family lived in to see patients; he only needed enough room to talk to patients, check their pulses and tongues, and prescribe herbal formulae or patent medicine. As his practice grew, he was able to rent another unit in the same apartment building to serve exclusively as his clinic.

There is a good number of practitioners of traditional Chinese medicine in the San Francisco Chinatown, and among them are pioneer practitioners who have practiced there for forty, fifty years; some even helped in the effort to have acupuncture legalized in the state of California. It did not take long for Gu Daifu to learn that he needed an acupuncture license in order to stay competitive in the field. He applied to one of the Chinese programs in the local TCM school. For two years, he worked five days a week and went to school over the weekends, twelve hours of classes on each day. He studied after clinic hours, and after he graduated from the master's program and passed the licensing exam, he chose to go on and attain a doctoral degree in Oriental Medicine. At the time, none of the local TCM schools in the Bay Area offered the doctoral level program, and the program he attended was an extension by an out-of-state school. Many of his teachers in the master's program became his classmates in the doctoral program, and in the end, many more Chinese practitioners with the OMD (Doctor of Oriental Medicine) degree were finally able to call themselves doctors again.

Now working with the acupuncture license, Gu Daifu feels much more confident practicing in America. He can claim insurance payments if his patients' health insurance plans cover the modality, which attracts some patients who cannot afford to pay out of their own pockets. In terms of his practice, it has not changed much. He still mostly prescribes herbs to treat his patients who come for his family's secret formulae. As an herbalist from a region in China where people were used to milder weather and had delicate palettes, his herbal tonics are less bitter and easier to swallow than most others.

When a patient walks into his clinic, she immediately sees Gu Daifu sitting behind his desk. He invites the patient to sit down and chitchat for a few minutes, for the patient to calm her breath and relax. He is known for being soft-spoken, polite, and very cautious in making his diagnoses.

On Gu Daifu's old office desk is a small velvet pillow for pulse reading. The patient rests one wrist on the pillow, and Gu Daifu quietly puts three fingers—the index, middle, and ring fingers of his right hand—across the patient's wrist. Almost like pressing chords on a guitar, he moves his fingers slightly and asserts pressure on different parts of the wrist to feel the movements of different meridians. After reading one wrist, he reads the other wrist as well. From the two wrists, he is able to determine the general conditions of all the meridians of the patient's body. He then asks the patient to stick out her tongue so that he can look at the color and appearance for further verification. The color of the facial complexion, the smell of the patient's breath, and the sound of her voice are also important sources of information regarding the patient's condition. He jots down notes on his chart, and shares his diagnosis with the patient while also asking whether she feels symptoms that are typical to the conditions that he identifies. Here is an example of how he explains to the patient while also trying to gather more information from the patient:

> It seems that there is not enough bodily fluid (*jinye* 津液) inside your body; essentially your body is now like a kettle boiling on the stove, but the water inside is drying up. Do you feel more thirsty than usual? Does your head feel warm or hurt?[6]

Gu Daifu has an extensive herbal dispensary in his clinic. Rather than displaying his herbs like the street-front herbal shops in Chinatown, his herbs are mostly hidden in his clinic, located on the fourth floor of a commercial building. After he designs an herbal formula for the patient, he walks behind a curtain by his desk, where there is a small space. Plastic drawers and recycled plastic containers filled with dried herbs stack against each other. He measures the herbs with a traditional lever and places them into small brown paper bags.

There are times when Gu Daifu prescribes patent medicine—mass-produced pills and honey chews containing popular and common formulae. Unlike herb packages that require brewing with water either on the stovetop or in a special herb kettle, patent medicine requires no preparation. The pills only need to be swallowed with some warm water. On the other hand, while the herb packages are customized according to the unique condition of each patient at the time of the clinic visit, patent medicine may not contain the most appropriate ingredients for the needs of the patient. Furthermore, some patent medicines contain herbs that are identified by the FDA as carcinogenic and are required by law to be labeled as such. Some patients refuse to take patent medicine after seeing the warning label; others feel compelled to ask more questions before they make informed decisions on what form of herbal formulae they choose.

In private, he acknowledges that acupuncture as a modality is still not his strength clinically, but his son, who just graduated from a chiropractic school, will be able to help him treat those patients who need manual treatments beyond herbal prescriptions.

Still speaking almost no English at all, Gu Daifu continues to work his way up the American social ladder. He invests in the American stock markets, and plans to purchase a house in the suburbs in the near future. "My son has grown," he exclaims excitedly, "and we must prepare him a house when he gets married and has kids."[7]

SU DAIFU: MANUAL HEALER[8]

Acupuncture, inserting needles by hand, belongs to the category of manual healing. However, there are many more manual techniques in traditional Chinese medicine; some require delicate tools and not so much force, such as acupuncture and cupping. Other techniques may require the healers to exert significant force to manually manipulate the patients' muscular-skeletal structure.

Zhenggu 整骨(or 正骨) and *tuina* 推拿 are two important specialties in traditional Chinese medicine, often labeled as Chinese orthopedics and Chinese massage, respectively. *Zhenggu* is similar to orthopedics in the way that it deals mostly with the muscular-skeletal structures and functions, but is in fact more similar to chiropractic and osteopathy in that it uses manual adjustments to treat pain caused by sprains, fractures, and injuries. *Tuina* is very closely related to *zhenggu*, but is indeed more similar to massage in that it focuses more on muscular treatments and very little on the bone structures. Some Chinese practitioners utilize a combination of both *zhenggu* and *tuina*, because while *zhenggu* can often treat twists and sprains very quickly by adjusting things back into their proper places, *tuina* is effective in relaxing muscle groups, which can serve as a helpful preparation for *zhenggu* treatments. Furthermore, patients seem to like the idea of getting a massage that takes more time but relaxes their muscles and relieves stress.

Often also practitioners and performers of martial arts, *zhenggu* and *tuina* practitioners were traditionally less educated than the herbal doctor literati and served the lower strata of the society. Some would travel from village to village to perform and provide manual treatments and simple herbal remedies for a living. In contemporary Chinese medicine, many of the techniques used by *zhenggu* and *tuina* are incorporated into orthopedic treatments and massage therapies. Traditional type practitioners can still be found serving Chinese communities all over the world, especially but not exclusively in rural areas with little medical resources.

Although there is no licensing requirement for *zhenggu* in California, and one can opt for the much less rigorous massage therapy certificate to practice *tuina*, the practitioners I know put themselves through the master's level TCM program and got licensed as acupuncturists. This was a practical move: in terms of social respect, the title of *zhongyi*, which many Chinese understand as the equivalent of a licensed acupuncturist in California, is much more respected than *zhenggu* or *tuina* practitioners, who are perceived as people who perform physical labor, and in the Chinese culture are considered one-tier below the *zhongyi* literati. On the financial front, licensed acupuncturists can claim health insurance payments whereas *zhenggu* or *tuina* masters cannot. Incidentally, both of the practitioners I know who practice exclusively *zhenggu* and *tuina* insist on being called "Doctor" (*yishi* or *daifu*), and appeared offended when addressed as "Master" (*shifu* 師傅).

When I first knew Su Daifu in 1999, he just immigrated to the Bay Area from Northern China. He was already practicing *zhenggu* to make a living, and had many patients who came by word of mouth. He was so skilled and effective in *zhenggu* that patients filled his tiny basement studio from 8:00 a.m. to 10:00 p.m., five days a week. There was barely any space between the folding massage table that he treated the patients on and the small couch that served somewhat as a waiting area. At night, after the patients were gone, the massage table doubled as his bed. The small couch was where he studied, and eventually he graduated from the TCM program and passed his acupuncture licensing exam.

Today, Su Daifu owns the building where his clinic is located. The first floor of the building is the clinic and has ten treatment rooms, which are constantly filled with patients. On the second floor are eight small rental units, and the rents he collects help pay for mortgage. Behind the building are a small garden and a cottage that he lives in. He is so pleased with his current life that he says, "If I could speak English, I would be really living the American dream."

It is actually amazing to see how Su Daifu, who knows no more than twenty words in English, runs a clinic where approximately 70 percent of his patients are non-Chinese. He has no hired assistance. When the phone rings, patients in the waiting room answer it for him. Those patients who can speak both English and Chinese translate phone conversations and sometimes even help interpret for patients who only speak English.

It is not easy talking "spirituality" with Su Daifu. He resists notions of religiosity (*zongjiao* 宗教), and like most Mainland Chinese practitioners in his generation, considers anything that is "unscientific" as "superstitious," which, to them, is almost like a dirty word used specifically against TCM practitioners. On the other hand, Su Daifu is an avid practitioner of *qigong*, who sees his personal *qigong* exercises as an integral part of his clinical treatments. Even after a twelve-hour day of treating patients, he still goes to the nearby school field at night to stretch, train, and cultivate his *qi*.

One day while he was treating a patient, I asked him why he found the *qigong* cultivation necessary, he replied, matter-of-factly:

> I work on these patients all day, how do you think I can handle that? Sometimes I don't even have time to eat. But you see, I rarely feel tired and sometime forget about hunger, because I do *qigong* to supply myself with the power (or strength; *liqi* 力氣) I need.

Su Daifu's nightly routine includes two hundred squat jumps, ten laps around the school track, and fifty pushups, followed by an almost *taichi*-like exercise that regenerates the ball of *qi* that encompasses his body. In his clinical treatments, he infuses *qi* into his patients if he feels it is necessary in addition to the purely manual techniques, especially when the treatment is not for purely muscular-skeletal problems, but involves massaging of the inner organs. He combines an extremely deep-pressing manual technique with infusion of *qi* directly into the inner organ.

To let me experience the sensation of such a method, he worked on my stomach for acid reflux, a condition that I've suffered for as long as I can remember. Like other *zhenggu* and *tuina* practitioners I know, Su Daifu treats all his patients with them fully clothed. His hands kneaded my stomach area, from a very light pressure and gradually deeper. After about three minutes, he pressed both of his thumbs directly into my stomach, so deep that I thought he was going to reach my spine. I let out a short scream. Then he infused *qi* into my stomach through his thumbs, which felt like something warm entering my stomach. The pressure was so intense that I stared at the white, plastered ceiling of the treatment room and thought I was about to die. Tears rolled down my cheeks uncontrollably. He smirked, as if he was thoroughly entertained by my reaction, and jokingly, yet perfectly, articulated his favorite word in English, "Relax ... relax ... "

It was one of the longest and most excruciating ten minutes in my life (another equally unforgettable incident was when another acupuncturist pierced two thin needles right through the sides of my nose). And when he finally released his thumbs, for a brief second I thought that part of my abdomen was never going to bounce back up and would stay permanently dented. But of course I survived to share the experience, and can attest that my abdomen was not deformed by the treatment. In fact, my acid reflux symptoms significantly lessened for about a week after the session.

It would be unfair to assume that one short treatment, although it felt to me like forever at the time, could cure a lifelong condition. However, his muscular-skeletal adjustments do have immediate and visible effects. For another treatment I underwent personally, he worked on my entire back to "straighten me up." I could not see what he was doing, but felt that he quickly loosened up the knots in the muscles. Nimbly (that was him) and painfully (that was me), he twisted, rolled, and pulled. It was very quick, taking about twenty minutes, from head to toe. At the same time, he was singing a song from his Cultural Revolution days, occasionally stopping to show me how to properly do the dance moves that went along with the song. I was very sore all over for about two days after the treatment, but "grew" about half an inch taller in height just from the one adjustment.

Besides *zhenggu* and *tuina*, Su Daifu also does acupuncture, cupping, and blood-letting depending on the needs of individual patients. He still believes that *zhenggu* and *tuina* are the most effective ways to treat most of the problems his patients come in with, but as his practice gets busier, acupuncture and cupping are much less labor-intensive. Furthermore, he can leave the patients in the treatment rooms with the needles in or cups on, and move on to treat other patients. This is not possible with *zhenggu* and *tuina*, although he also has his interns work on new patients or do the *tuina* part of the treatments before he comes in for the *zhenggu*.

ALBERT: RITUAL HEALER[9]

Healing illnesses by incantations, making and burning of talismans, and other rituals that drove away unwanted or evil spirits had always been one branch of Chinese medicine. Classically identified as *zhuyouke* 祝由科 (specialization in rituals and incantations), ritual healing was an important alternative to herbal prescriptions.[10] As the Communist Chinese government aggressively removed all elements of "superstition" from the standardized TCM, *zhuyouke* is no longer part of the regulated medical profession in China. However, healers who utilize rituals and/or other spiritual tools to expel diseases can still be found in Chinese communities.

Albert is in his forties, pale and timid, and often has a touch of nervousness in his voice. In the ten years since he migrated to the Bay Area from Mainland China, Albert has been known by the local Chinese community mostly as a skillful master in *fengshui* 風水.[11] In fact, I got to know Albert a few years ago because he wanted to translate a book he had written on *fengshui* from Chinese to English. After several honest discussions, the project fell through. Still a new immigrant at the time, Albert had very little contact with non-Chinese, and rarely ventured outside of the Chinese-dense neighborhoods. As a result, he was not yet aware of the fact that the cultural gap between China and California was beyond geographic distance, and beyond just the languages. His book was an excellent compilation of *fengshui* cases that he had encountered and solved, but the content assumed that the readers have a relatively high competency in general *fengshui* concepts and Chinese cultural knowledge. In my opinion, if the book were to be translated literally and directly from the original, the general American readers would probably find it difficult to understand.

Rather than being offended by my frank analysis, Albert kept in touch and remained a friend. When we occasionally meet for a cup of tea or to share a meal, Albert tells me about his life stories, not just as a *fengshui* master, but also as a fortune teller/astrologer (*mingli shi* 命理師), an esoteric Daoist ritualist, a *qigong* teacher, and a practicing acupuncturist. Of all the practitioners I know, he comes closest to a classical *zhuyouke* healer.

When I first knew Albert, he was already enrolled in one of the TCM schools in the Bay Area. The student visa issued by the school allowed him to stay in the United States while attending the program. He provided *fengshui* consultations and fortune telling services to other Chinese immigrants and diasporans, and quickly expanded his clientele to include non-Chinese as well. His English skills improved rapidly, and with the steady growth of his one-man business, he became financially comfortable and socially established. After graduating from the TCM program and attaining his California acupuncture license, he found connections to change his foreign student status into permanent residency.

Given the many hats that he wears professionally, Albert has an interesting scope of practice. He provides most services out of the small rental apartment he lives in, and does house visits for *fengshui* consultations upon request. Interestingly, as Albert's repertoire of practices grows, he decreased his usage of Daoist magic and rituals significantly. I asked him why he now avoids using magic and rituals, and he explained:

> Rituals and magic that change the natural flow of things will eventually backfire. If you help somebody else interrupt the natural flow of things, it affects your own flow in life.

He goes on to share an example,

> I have these two friends, a married couple. The husband was having affairs, and the wife came to me to ask for a talisman that would get her husband back. She added burnt talisman ashes into the coke he drank at every meal. She said, you know, he's been very good, comes home on time and actually helps around the house, just that he seems a little aloof. Then the husband went on to a business trip, and because the wife didn't go along and didn't give him more burnt talisman, the magic wore off and he started having affairs again. So at the end it didn't work out anyway, and people took longer to get to where they were supposed to get to in the first place. Most important of all, because I helped the wife on doing it, I seemed to have more obstacles in my own life than usual during that time period. So I don't do the talismans anymore because it makes my own life worse.[12]

Albert's perspective is actually consistent with the other Chinese folk and Daoist ritualists I have talked to. The belief, which is often supported by the practitioners' own personal experiences, is that there seems to be a real energetic transaction when a magic or a ritual is performed to change the natural flow of an event or a situation. If a negative experience is understood as some kind of energetic attack, then by performing a magic or a ritual to help a client avoid the attack, now the attack is redirected toward the ritualist instead. The attack could take form of accidents that result in physical injuries, strange but frequent obstacles in everyday life, and sudden illnesses that medical professionals find hard to explain.

Albert, who is also a clairvoyant, can actually see the negative energies, sometimes in the form of ghostly apparitions and other monstrous or grotesque entities. I have seen him refuse to enter a treatment room in another practitioner's clinic where he already saw that an entity was attached to the patient. He practically leaped backward to get away, and there was real fear in his eyes. He said that the entity looked like a giant glob of mucus that completely covered the patient's face, and he was too afraid to go close to it. The patient was seeking treatment for a severe case of congestion and sinus pain.

In order to protect himself from these energetic attacks that are sometimes inevitable, Albert practices *qigong* diligently. He even does different forms of *qigong* cultivations to compare their effectiveness, and sometimes teaches to his clients who are interested. After experimenting with two different *qigong* forms, one from the Buddhist tradition and another from the Daoist tradition, he shares:

> People who do the Buddhist practices, especially those who talk about giving and spreading goodwill, tend to be fatter because their *qi*

spreads more outward. They don't *shougong*收功 [a finishing movement to end a sequence and keep the *qi* inside the body], so their *qi* is always just out there. On the other hand, people who practice Daoist cultivation that focus on accumulating *qi* and building *neidan*內丹 [inner elixir] are thin. It actually makes people lose weight, and they lose weight very quickly. I've tried both ways. So when I did the Buddhist cultivation, very quickly I became visibly fatter, face rounder and my flesh felt filled. Then I started doing Daoist *qigong* and lost a lot of weight. My face became narrow and muscles became tighter. There were two clients who practiced *qigong* with me, and within weeks they both lost weight.[13]

Before I have a chance to point out the commercial implications of the weight-loss effects of the Daoist *qigong*, Albert quickly adds: "But people gain the weight back if they don't keep on practicing. It's about practice and persistence... very scientific."

Albert is not alone in considering TCM healing practices first and foremost as "scientific." He argues that Chinese astrology, which he utilizes for both *fengshui* consultation and fortune telling, is based heavily on statistics and thousands of years of human experience. And to him, nothing is more scientific and less superstitious than something that is based on statistics and practiced by calculations.

RECAP: TCM IN THE CHINESE DIASPORA

The practitioners in this chapter demonstrate some variations of how TCM is practiced in Chinese community in the Bay Area. In the context of the Chinese diaspora, these practitioners are simultaneously negotiating their roles in several systems. Geographically located in California and under the jurisdiction of the state's legal system, the practitioners are quick to find that a state license for acupuncture grants them some medical authority, access to health insurance coverage for their services, and eligibility for malpractice insurance that protects them in case of lawsuits from patients. As members of the Chinese ethnic community, they legitimate their professional authority by the means of acupuncture licenses, but offer services to meet the demands of the Chinese diasporans in their expectations for medical plurality and technical specializations within TCM.

Two generations of Linda's family offer acupuncture services in the Bay Area. Linda's father not only provides care to the low-income sector of the Chinatown population, he charges them much lower than practitioners outside of Chinatown, and accepts MediCal patients who would otherwise not be able to afford not only acupuncture, but any kind of healthcare at all. Her aunt and uncle not only treat patients using acupuncture and herbs, they also participate in social and political movements promoting acknowledgment of and justice for TCM practitioners. Linda is the first in the family to venture outside of the Chinese community. Like other TCM practitioners who serve mostly non-Chinese clienteles, Linda has a long road ahead of her in educating her patients about TCM, and acquiring a large enough client base to sustain the practice.

Gu Daifu, Su Daifu, and Albert treat patients with non-acupuncture modalities that their Chinese ethnic patients are familiar with. The non-acupuncture specializations provide practitioners a competitive edge in the Chinese ethnic consumer market. There is a cultural understanding that practitioners with different specializations are good for specific types of health concerns. For example, one may choose to visit a manual healer for muscular-skeletal adjustments, an herbalist for flu symptoms and general conditioning, and an acupuncturist for pain management. That is not to say that any of these modalities are ineffective for other types of complaints, but one may choose to use each mode of practice most efficiently. Patients who find one modality insufficient to treat the problem may try another modality, then another, then another. It is very similar to temple-hopping, which is common in Chinese societies; it is considered beneficial to establish connections widely so that a variety of resources are available in different times of need.

NOTES

1. See http://www.lhc.ca.gov/studies/175/UCSFscope.pdf (accessed April 8, 2009).
2. Ibid.
3. Personal interview with Linda, September 24, 2008. Interview was conducted entirely in English.
4. PRC here stands for People's Republic of China. See introduction for more on PRC-TCM.
5. Informal interviews and interactions with Gu Daifu were conducted entirely in mandarin Chinese, and quotes were translated into English by the author.
6. Clinic observation, June 5, 2009.
7. Personal communication, October 7, 2009.
8. Informal interviews and interactions with Su Daifu were conducted entirely in mandarin Chinese, and quotes translated into English by author.
9. Personal interviews on March 15, 2008 and September 9, 2008. Interviews were conducted entirely in Mandarin Chinese, and quotes were translated into English by the author.
10. For historical study of classical *zhuyouke* healers, see dissertation by Philip S. Cho, *Ritual and the Occult in Chinese Medicine and Religious Healing: The Development of Zhuyou Exorcism* (University of Pennsylvania, 2005).
11. *Fengshui*, often also known as geomancy, is an ancient Chinese art in selecting ideal locations and directional orientations for residences, businesses, and graves.
12. Personal interview, September 9, 2008.
13. Personal interview, March 15, 2008.

FIVE
TCM as Complementary Medicine

Starting with this chapter, we will see more of how TCM practitioners in the Bay Area conceptualize, orient, and realize their healing practices in the ambiguous area between biomedicine and holistic medicine, between Chinese and American mainstream cultures, between their personal beliefs and market demands. It is a matrix where each practitioner is uniquely located in the mix and where fixed categories fail to sufficiently cover the possibilities. The care for a spiritual dimension of human existence is an important ongoing dialogue among practitioners and patients, but not everyone is equally enthusiastic about it. However, the pervasiveness of the interest and demand for spiritual-related care in itself becomes an issue to which the practitioners must respond or at least react. Viewed as favorable for the profession by some and unfavorable by others, the spiritual dimension of TCM practices becomes a pivotal point in how the practitioners orient themselves.

The practitioners we meet in this chapter work within the biomedical institutions using TCM to complement biomedical treatments. Already accepted as members of the biomedical community, whether by previous training in biomedicine or recognition as specialists in acupuncture as a treatment modality, they work very closely with biomedical doctors, often alongside them on creating comprehensive treatment plans for patients.

THOMAS (MD WITH PRIVATE ACUPUNCTURE PRACTICE)[1]

Thomas greets me in his office on a Monday; he usually does not see patients on Mondays. With tanned skin and donning a cheerful Hawaiian shirt, Thomas's appearance and light-spirited character makes him look more like a vacationer in the Bahamas than a doctor at work, granted it is his day off. He works four days in the week, and sees an average of twenty patients a day.[2] "I figure that's enough money and I only need so much money," Thomas explains. "If I work more than that I burn out."

Thomas is the only U.S.-trained biomedical physician among the practitioners in this study. His clinic is located in a medical complex that is closely affiliated with the teaching medical center across the street, where he once did his internal medicine residency as a newly minted MD.

The year was 1973, and Thomas went to England on a holiday. There he fell in love with a woman who introduced him to acupuncture. A young doctor with true passion for medicine and healing, Thomas decided to stay in London for more training in acupuncture. After all, he smirked, "If it worked out, great, if not I just come back and do regular medicine. I had a good backup plan." The enthusiastic couple and their friends pooled together money to pay any good acupuncturist they could find in London. Without a formal "school" or credential, they sought acupuncturists with a wide range of styles, and invited those who went to China to learn new techniques to talk to the group. "It was a wonderful thing!" he reminisces.

This was when acupuncture was still a controversial modality both in Europe and the United States, and traditional Chinese medicine was not yet widely known outside of the Chinese ethnic community. In the United Kingdom, the public ignorance of TCM actually provided freedom and abundant resources:

> The government there had the attitude that acupuncture was so ridiculous we don't have to have any regulations at all. As a result, the true laissez-faire of all kinds, good stuff, weird stuff, stuff that I would call bad, all kinds. There were many styles you can pick and choose and see, and to realize that there are many ways of doing something.

Thomas turned thirty in 1975, and decided that he had to do something with his life. He decided to start an acupuncture clinic back in the Bay Area and see if he could make a living with what he learned in London. He was quick to utilize his credentials and connections as a biomedical physician to his benefit. Other physicians in the medical center, many of whom Thomas did his residency with, referred their patients to him. Even if they were not sure about acupuncture or TCM, they trusted Thomas and his biomedical training. Thomas did not disappoint his physician friends and the patients who came to him. His clinic was a success since the beginning.

The way Thomas runs through the list of problems he treats the most in his clinic reminds me of a frontier doctor, a physician who would be the only physician in a few hundred miles, who has to treat everything under the sun:

> Things I see most of the times . . . let me see. Back problems. Back pain, neck pain, all different etiologies, headaches, allergies, and asthma.

> Women with menstrual and hormonal things. Other joint problems, and skin, and a fair number of psychological problems . . . anxiety and depression. A lot of weird things that people can't figure them out, or they don't heal the way they ought to. A lot of people with multiple sclerosis, people with strokes. . . . It's a general practice of everything. Really everything you can think of.

The fact is, of course, Thomas practices in a community with probably the highest concentration of biomedical healthcare providers in the Bay Area. He is aware that his practice is unique even for a family physician, and that his cross-disciplinarity is ambiguously and delicately positioned. For example, although he can legitimately order laboratory tests for his patients, he rarely does so. Instead, he would encourage his patients to go back to their "regular physicians" or family physicians. "Hey, these guys refer patients to me," he points out, "I don't want to make them feel like I'm taking their customers away. Let's all work together and I want to keep everybody happy."

Similarly, although Thomas sometimes performs acupuncture on his patients' pets, he does it as a hobby and never charges them for the treatments. "I can treat animals like a good Samaritan," he explains, "but I don't want to get the veterinarians upset."

On the other hand, where he is able to provide what other biomedical physicians cannot, Thomas provides with little reservation. His total medicine not only seems to cover a wide range of concerns, he also tries to care for different dimensions of his patients' lives:

> [M]aybe I didn't totally fix your back, but your general attitude toward life is better, and you sleep better. It's like a lot of times a person is better off, but the thing they came for isn't better. Or it can be the other way around. I prefer to see, perhaps I didn't fix the particular thing you came for, but really your life is smoother and easier. The way to describe acupuncture is that it's like a tune-up and oil change. I think that's the best metaphor I've come up with. Another one is, sometimes I'd say this, a tune-up and oil change for your self-repair mechanism.

He further explains the psychological and many other dimensions of his practice:

> First of all, you don't make a distinction. You would say psychological, physical, just different perspectives of the same thing. [Gets out of his chair.] So from this side I see you, and I move around [dashes to the other side of the room] . . . it's physical right, I walk over here, it's economic problem, or it's, oh, spiritual. It's one thing, but our language makes it divide into pieces. Then we forget that it's not pieces. It's useful to analyze it, and it's useful to break them into pieces, but you should never forget that it's really just one thing. So you never make these distinctions between psychological. For the sake of discussion we can say, gee, you know, this seems like you have a lot of grief in your life.

He gives an example:

> So this guy, an artist who was just in here in the last few weeks, he has etiopathic pulmonary fibrosis, which is like an untreatable lung disease. I was just talking to him. In Chinese medicine you say, lungs, grief. Anxiety and grief . . . how does that affect your life? How long have you had this illness? So, my wife, you know, we had this wonderful marriage for many years, she just died quickly, and this started a few months later. I told him that, just knowing that connection, the lungs and grief, it's the same thing. You can say it's caused by this intense grief, but you can also say, it's just, it is the same. It is the same imbalance in the universe.

Whereas one might expect a biomedical physician practicing acupuncture to have advantages in the biomedical-framed insurance system, Thomas actually perceives himself in a disadvantageous position against dominating TCM standards:

> Usually [my patients] are in for an hour, and I spend twenty to thirty minutes with the patient. It's a long time, and I can do my time as a [biomedical] doctor. [Health insurances and Workers Compensation cover acupuncture treatments], but they want you to do it a certain way. They want you to do three treatments a week. Well, you can do that. I almost never do that. I like to see people once a week or even less than that. If you wait, you get a whole lot more information. . . . If they are better, I go that direction. If they are not better, usually that means I was wrong, and I should go a different direction, start it over. I do that three times.
>
> You get at least double the information by waiting a little bit. You gotta wait. But the people who designed the insurance code did it one way, and that's what they want you to do. I have to go to them and say, I want to do less treatments. Or let me do the same number of treatments but spread out. Each time I have to fight. They are so used to one style, they don't realize that there are many styles.

Thomas is quite insistent on practicing in a way that makes sense to him, even if it means diverting from the perceived norm of TCM:

> There is a big variation in how exactly the needles should go into the points. Some do it this way and that way. Some take the pulse and some don't. I mostly don't take the pulse; I can, but mostly I don't. There is a huge spectrum of what people do and can do.

Perhaps this is what integrative medicine should really look like—a hybrid between medical systems that allows the practitioners to better understand their patients in every way. One popular approach favored by health insurance companies and biomedical institutions is to incorporate TCM modalities into the biomedical conceptual framework. Thomas allows himself freedom to venture between the two:

Traditional Chinese medicine is great because it gives you some tools, ladders ... intellectual ladders to move from one level to another. It's a very powerful thing. It's powerful even if you were going to use Western medicine to treat them. Thinking in this Chinese medicine's way, you could get some good insight in what's going on.

CHRIS (LICENSED ACUPUNCTURIST WORKING FOR BIOMEDICAL ESTABLISHMENT)[3]

On a sunny afternoon, I walk into a biomedical establishment that provides its patients with acupuncture services. Chris opened his office door to greet me. If it were not for the "L.Ac." (Licensed Acupuncturist) embroidered onto his white clinical coat, no one would be able to distinguish Chris from the biomedical physicians who work in the same clinic. A Caucasian American man in his forties, Chris comes across as confident and intellectual. Chris has ended his own private practice as he phases into the current arrangement of working for the biomedical establishment full-time.

Chris's entry point was *Aikido* 合氣道, a Japanese martial art form. The practice of *Aikido* not only took Chris to Japan, where he lived for some time in his younger years, the martial art also introduced acupuncture treatments to him. Life then took Chris back to the United States, and he landed in California. He started a career in bodywork, and worked as a massage therapist to support himself until he graduated from one of the local TCM schools in 2000. He also completed a six-month internship in China, where "the number of patients they see in one morning is more than what we see in the school clinics here in an entire semester."

Having worked as a solo practitioner and now for the biomedical establishment, Chris is keen to compare the two vastly different models. Unlike in a private practice, an acupuncturist who works for the biomedical establishment is not considered a primary care provider, but a pain management specialist who also takes patients who suffer from side effects of chemotherapy. More specifically, whereas private acupuncturists usually see and treat a wide range of conditions, Chris sees only referrals from inside the biomedical establishment. His patients have already been assessed and diagnosed by general physicians and specialists, and are only referred to him if they request acupuncture for pain management and chemotherapy-related conditions, and/or if their physicians feel that acupuncture can be helpful. The biomedical establishment also limits its acupuncturists to treating only chronic pain and with only needles. In other words, Chris does not treat patients with short-term or acute pain, and does not utilize modalities outside of needling, such as cupping and herbs that are commonly used in private practices. Furthermore, because the patients come to Chris already with diagnoses, he only treats them for the specific conditions that they are referred to him for, and nothing more.

Working under the biomedical establishment guarantees Chris's patient base, and Chris no longer has to worry about marketing, health insurance claims, and fee collection. The biomedical establishment has a well-established computer database where Chris schedules patient appointments and accesses patient information and medical records. As a result, Chris has no paperwork or any kind of paper clutter. Furthermore, the establishment's large patient base gives Chris twenty patients in a full day of work, where Chris works eight-hour days and sees three to four patients simultaneously in any given time block. On average, he spends five to ten minutes on patient intake and interview, and ten to forty minutes on the actual acupuncture, depending on the needs of individual patients.

When Chris sees a patient, he has a moving lamp station that has a stereo boom box tied to the stand, on which Chris plays for his patients his collection of soothing, calming music, primarily New Age compositions with Indian, Hindu, Chinese, and Japanese elements and sounds. With a background in bodywork, Chris feels it is important to create the proper ambience. Patients mostly enjoy relaxing to his music collection. However, if the patients wish to listen to their own music, he welcomes them to play any type of music they prefer. Since he sees patients in all age groups, there have been times when teenage patients bring in gangster rap or popular country music. "If listening to the music they like and are familiar with can make them less anxious about the needles," Chris chuckles, "I guess that is still helpful."

Chris admits that he sometimes has his own diagnoses on his patients' conditions from the perspective of traditional Chinese medicine. During the treatment session, he often engages the patients in how the system of traditional Chinese medicine differs from biomedicine, and how he may have a different perspective on their conditions. He also has handouts for patients who are interested in learning more about acupuncture or traditional Chinese medicine.

Working alongside biomedical health providers has also been a positive experience for Chris. He learned that the biomedical establishment has been in internal discussion for the past twenty-five years on alternative treatments and integrative possibilities. On the individual level, he has found the biomedical physicians he encounters in the establishment to be genuinely interested in learning more about traditional Chinese medicine. It came as a surprise, because that was inconsistent with the picture that was painted for him during his school training:

> In school we were taught that we are different and alternative, and offer what the Western MDs don't offer. There were a lot of cultural stereotypes that could have been misunderstandings. I've come to

learn that Western medicine is more open-minded toward TCM than TCM is toward Western medicine.

Chris's close working relationship with biomedical physicians also gives him exposure to the circle of medical acupuncturists, who are biomedical physicians practicing acupuncture or incorporating acupuncture into their biomedical practices. Since the biomedical physicians can legally practice invasive clinical procedures, they are not required to attain a state acupuncture license to utilize acupuncture in their clinical practices. Most licensed acupuncturists have neither interactions nor relationships with medical acupuncturists. Moreover, some licensed acupuncturists accuse the medical acupuncturists of using acupuncture without proper understanding of the framework of traditional Chinese medicine. Chris begs to differ:

> Some medical acupuncturists really want to learn TCM beyond just inserting the needles. Their symposiums are fantastic. I have met and known a few who are very versed in TCM principles and always want to learn more.

On the other hand, Chris finds the continuing education courses for the licensed acupuncturists unsatisfactory, if not downright embarrassing:

> Sometimes the classes are like infomercials, and lack good substance. Some instructors sell their notes for ridiculous fees. They remind me of travelling medicine shows, where they sell secret elixirs from one small town to the next.

In addition, Chris is critical of those practitioners who try to attach spirituality to the medicine. He adheres to the view that, contrary to common conception, TCM was born around the time of the Cultural Revolution and was an attempt of the Chinese Communist Party to compile traditional medical theories and practices in order to educate the barefoot doctors and export to the West. As a recently reinvented medicine that was intentionally packaged to be practical, Chris asserts, revival or reinsertion of the spiritual aspect of the medicine is not necessarily helpful. It becomes clear that his criticism is mainly targeted toward the Caucasian or non-Chinese practitioners:

> Very few graduates from the TCM programs make it to the profession, because American acupuncture students often have certain assumptions or preconceptions before coming in. But New Age movement is not synonymous with TCM, and practicing TCM doesn't make one a Daoist either. What keeps acupuncturists in the ball game of the profession is actually more about looking professional and having the patients take them seriously.

Chris shares his own working model:

TCM is a medicine, and my own spirituality shouldn't matter. Different philosophies can coexist, and I am personally eclectic. TCM should be about convenience and practicality, where we can always add more. It is also important to keep an open mind and be culturally sensitive, because I work with a very diverse demographic. And to work in the [biomedical establishment], it is crucial to understand Western diagnoses, whereas most TCM program graduates don't come with that. I think the doctoral programs offered by the TCM schools are trying to make up that gap.

KELLY (LICENSED ACUPUNCTURIST WORKING FOR AN INTEGRATIVE MEDICINE CENTER IN A BIOMEDICAL TEACHING HOSPITAL AND WITH A NON-PROFIT CLINIC FOR UNDERPRIVILEGED WOMEN)[4]

The clinic assistant lets me know that Kelly is still with a patient, and I settle into the waiting area. As I sit down on the couch, I notice the luxury of a well-funded medical center: not luxury in terms of being served caviar and champagne, but the luxury of a high-ceiling, spacious, well-lit waiting area in a clinic situated in the heart of one of the most expensive cities in the world. I can faintly hear the assistant answering phone calls and clicking on her computer keyboard; it is a distance close enough where I feel accessible to help but far enough to not be distracted. The couch is obviously carefully chosen; it is comfortable and ergonomically supportive at the same time. A range of popular magazines are neatly fanned out on the coffee table.

This is the Integrative Medicine Center in one of the most prestigious teaching medical centers in the nation. More than half of the practitioners working in this clinic have biomedical training and credentials: they are physicians, psychiatrists, nurses, and midwives who integrate alternative and complementary medicines with biomedicine; many of the MDs are also on the teaching faculty of the affiliated medical school. The rest of the practitioners, who are without biomedical credentials, are yoga and meditation instructors, massage therapists, acupuncturists, and biofeedback practitioners. The center also trains resident physicians (MDs) who are interested in practicing medicine in a way that

> emphasizes the combination of both conventional and alternative approaches to address the biological, psychological, social and spiritual aspects of health and illness. It emphasizes respect for the human capacity for healing, the importance of the relationship between the practitioner and the patient, a collaborative approach to patient care among practitioners, and the practice of conventional, complementary, and alternative health care that is evidence-based.[5]

The Integrative Medicine Center's location—directly across the street from the world-renowned Oncology Center that takes up the entire street block—hints at its focus on oncology-related care. The focus is also clearly indicated by the past and ongoing evidence-based research projects conducted by the researchers in this center.

Kelly first became involved with the Integrative Medicine Center to participate in a research project that looked at the effect of acupuncture and herbs on women with breast cancer. On the breast-cancer floor in the Oncology Center, Kelly practiced acupuncture on the patients alongside biomedical physicians and clinical researchers. At the time, she was also quite occupied with her own private practice and a non-profit community clinic for low-income women that she cofounded. The director of the Integrative Medicine Center consulted her on expanding the team of clinical practitioners in the center, hoping that she would help them in hiring trustworthy and capable acupuncturists to join the team. After many rounds of resume reviews and discussions, Kelly liked the search committee so much that she joined the team herself, and eventually chose to end her private practice completely. Her work with the non-profit clinic continues. The clinic is run by female volunteers and provides acupuncture, herbal medicine, homeopathy, massage, and social work services to low-income, underprivileged women with cancer. In short, between her two jobs Kelly provides care to patients who have abundant financial and social resources, and also patients with very little financial and social resources.

Kelly is finally able to see me. She leads me through the clinic hallway decorated with bamboo screen and live evergreen vines, and finds an empty treatment room where we could both sit down. Still short of breath from a busy morning, she sits down by an Asian-style cabinet, and opens up a small microwave container. Kelly has only a small block of time to talk with me while a patient rests with acupuncture needles inserted, and the time also triple-duties as lunch break.

Since a very young age, Kelly had always wanted to be a physician of some sort. She majored in biology and chemistry in college, and was interested in eventually furthering her education in biomedicine. Then during the third year of her undergraduate study, Kelly lost her mother to a surgery. The personal tragedy took Kelly away from school for a year. In that year she explored ways to heal, and encountered a naturopathy practitioner who incorporated acupuncture into her practice. Fascinated by the alternative healing practices, Kelly asked if the practitioner could teach her.

As Kelly finished her undergraduate work and later entered acupuncture school, she always followed and worked with her naturopathic mentor. However, Kelly does not incorporate homeopathy in her practice at all. Her integration is predominantly between TCM and biomedicine, with TCM in the foreground:

> I want to create a diagnosis that's a TCM diagnosis and [I tell the patients] that's how I'm going to treat them. Now I might have a knowing that if you are on this type of chemotherapy drug the likelihood of it having this outcome and creating these different blood deficiencies or . . . having an understanding of what's going to happen with that. My knowledge of biomedical system is important because it makes the patient feel better, and it has nothing to do with how I'm choosing treatment. And I will absolutely tell them what I want to know: what drugs they are on, what type of cancer they have.
>
> [It is important to] have a TCM diagnosis . . . the value is that it makes [the patients] more comfortable and it feels safer in the process, and also potentially being able to have a good idea of when something is going wrong and have them address it. [I would say, for example,] I think that something is changing with your liver function and I would like for you to go get some blood work, or I'd like for you to get an ultrasound.

Her familiarity with the biomedical system also seems to contribute to her confidence in working with biomedical physicians:

> I think one of the things that I believe [the TCM] profession does, is very often it becomes defensive. We should be really comfortable about being questioned, and we should be comfortable about questioning back. I don't recommend chemotherapy, but I certainly talk to all of my patients about their treatment regimes, and I talk to them about how they should talk to their oncologists. And I feel comfortable with their oncologists talking to me.

She admits that the oncologists usually include TCM in developing a treatment plan only upon the request of the patients. In other words, TCM treatments, and acupuncture in particular, is not a routine component of an oncology treatment plan there. However, if the patients decide that it might be helpful to include TCM, then Kelly or one of her licensed acupuncturist colleagues at the Integrative Medicine Center would be invited to participate in designing the treatment plan.

Utilizing the two systems side by side can be very helpful, but Kelly also expresses her frustration with oversimplified and universalized translations across systems:

> I don't like it when people [say] you have a disease that's defined in biomedicine, [therefore] all those people's organs have the same TCM diagnosis, and they should all be treated the same. That's why research [for efficacy of TCM treatments] is so difficult—because [the cases are] individualized and it should be, and the diagnoses don't translate [across systems].

Over the past few years working in the Integrative Medicine Center, she noticed changes in the demographics of her patients that indicate increased inclusion of her services as part of oncology care. At first, she saw mostly patients at the end of their lives; gradually she saw more and more patients before they had surgery or chemotherapy. In other words, TCM has become incorporated into the treatment plans earlier and more extensively. Often the referrals come not from the patients' physicians, but also from friends and nurses who heard or knew about acupuncture treatments.

However, she thinks much of the trust from her MD colleagues seem to be for her personally, which does not necessarily extend to TCM in general or other TCM practitioners:

> I think there is still bias [against TCM in general]. The oncologists here, many of them would feel comfortable with people seeing me, but not somebody else that would do exactly the very same thing. I think that bias is just based on because they know me. It's just interesting—they'll often ask me what do I think about herbs that someone else prescribes or something like that but the referral piece is much more expansive than it used to be. They are much more comfortable with it.

In a research hospital with an evidence-based approach, it is interesting to hear that on the personal level, physicians still place more trust on non-biomedical practitioners they know personally.

When I ask Kelly about her perspective on how the spiritual and spiritual cultivations relate to her clinical practice, she shares:

> I do exercise. I have some depth of experience in *Taichi*. I want to be— so I've taken it for many years but be very clear that I think we in the [United] States don't have a particularly good understanding of the depth of knowledge that that really requires for you to be able to engage in a way that's comprehensive helping you physically, mentally, spiritually so that's more related to the medicine and what I incorporate in my life.

RECAP: THE POWER OF BIOMEDICINE

Although Thomas, Chris, and Kelly came to TCM from different entry points and professional training, they currently locate squarely within the biomedical system, where biomedical physicians view them as specialists and respected colleagues. Unlike many TCM practitioners who provide healthcare without having much cooperative relationships or even direct contacts with biomedical physicians, these practitioners work alongside biomedical physicians. As part of the biomedical cohort, these practitioners are endorsed by the biomedical community as trustworthy practitioners. Such endorsement brings patient referrals from biomedical practitioners, opportunities to conduct research projects funded by biomedical institutions, and respect from patients and other TCM practitioners.

With Thomas, who was trained as a biomedical physician in the United States before he explored TCM in England, the biomedical credential automatically exempted him from having to obtain an acupuncture license. For many pioneer practitioners who practiced TCM before there were TCM training programs in the Bay Area or legal regulations for acupuncture in California, the licensing system eventually grandfathered them in. For TCM practitioners who have no other medical credentials, being licensed for acupuncture is the only way for them to claim insurance payments or acquire malpractice insurance. Thomas weighed his options and found that, for him, claiming insurance payments as a family physician was easier than claiming them as an acupuncturist. The freedom to access both medical systems provides options; therefore, Thomas can take advantage of both of his professional identities to optimize convenience and possibly monetary gain as well. Even if a patient has a health insurance plan that does not cover acupuncture treatments, Thomas can still claim for his services under office visits as a biomedical physician.

Furthermore, the peer relationship with other biomedical physicians in the community remained active and strong even when he came back to the United States with a new medical paradigm in tow. Those physicians who had worked with Thomas when he was an intern in the biomedical teaching hospital had confidence in his medical skills and judgment. On the other hand, Thomas is careful to maintain friendly relationships with his biomedical colleagues by referring patients back to their biomedical physicians for laboratory tests, even though he can order laboratory tests as well. The positioning of himself as a professionally competent peer who offers services that complement regular biomedical practices (rather than competing against them) has proven to be successful.

Chris is positioned within the biomedical establishment as a pain management specialist who exclusively uses acupuncture. He does not practice the full scope of practice legally allowed for licensed acupuncturists in California because the institutional arrangement does not allow Chris to utilize other TCM modalities or make independent diagnoses. On the other hand, the institution provides him with financial stability and full administrative support.

There are several advantages to Chris's position. First, the physicians in the biomedical institution can only refer patients to acupuncturists within the institution. Not only does that guarantee Chris a full schedule of treatment sessions, but also the patients who may otherwise have no access to acupuncture treatments are now offered the option. In his interactions with patients, Chris educates his patients on TCM preventive and conditioning strategies, such as specific exercises and lifestyle tips. This helps promote TCM to a broader spectrum of the general population that independent TCM practitioners may not be able to reach. Chris also enjoys the intellectual exchanges as a member of the cohort of biomedical physicians. Not only does he learn from these colleagues about the biomedical perspective and approaches on healthcare, he also offers the

TCM perspective and strategies to physicians who are interested in learning more.

Kelly is well known in the Bay Area for her work with the Integrative Medical Center and the non-profit community clinic. As a practitioner in a prestigious teaching medical center, where she is directly involved in defining the standard and expectations for TCM practitioners, she is respected by the biomedical community. As a result, she has better access to personal networks and social resources only available to accepted members of this elite cohort of biomedical physicians. For example, since the non-profit clinic relies on grants and donor funding, Kelly's position as a practitioner and researcher at the Integrative Medical Center is likely to increase donor confidence to invest in the clinic.

It is important to note that all three above practitioners view themselves and their biomedical colleagues as equals in the same intellectual cohort. Their personal influences on those biomedical practitioners who work with them can be profound. The trust they cultivate in their biomedical colleagues, even if the trust is mainly in them as individuals, is a crucial start for communication between medical systems.

NOTES

1. Personal interview, April 28, 2008. The interview was conducted in English.
2. The average of twenty patients per day and eighty patients per week is more than most TCM practitioners I include in this study. Unlike the few extremely popular practitioners who have interns and assistants, clinics with multiple practitioners, and school clinics, solo practitioners with no assistants typically see no more than ten patients per working day. Some practitioners simply do not have large enough patient bases to see more than three to four patients in a working day. Thomas equates his clinic to a typical family physician practice, and claims that for his practice to be sustainable long-term, he needs to have at least three thousand patients on file.
3. Personal interview, October 14, 2008. The interview was conducted in English.
4. Personal interview, August 12, 2008. The interview was conducted in English.
5. See Osher Center for Integrative Medicine website http://www.osher.ucsf.edu/about/integrativemed.html (accessed October 8, 2009).

SIX
TCM as an Alternative Medicine

Unlike those who want to provide for what biomedicine lacks and are content working within the biomedical system, some practitioners are dissatisfied with the biomedical system and aim to provide services alternative to biomedicine. These two modes—as complementary to biomedicine and as alternative to biomedicine—both play off biomedicine as the standard and dominant mode of medicine.

In this chapter, we hear from the practitioners who view themselves as medical professionals who offer patients an alternative to biomedicine. Unlike the previous group of practitioners, who work within the biomedical system or even on the same teams as the biomedical physicians, the practitioners in this group view TCM as a medical system that is parallel to biomedicine rather than integrated into the biomedical system.

JOY AND ADAM (LICENSED ACUPUNCTURISTS IN PRIVATE PRACTICE; TCM SCHOOL ADMINISTRATOR AND PROFESSORS)[1]

Joy is Chinese American, and Adam is Caucasian American. They are both licensed acupuncturists. Not only does the married couple share a practice, they often finish each other's sentences. Extremely enthusiastic about their work, they both speak with breakneck speed and roll their words into long, unpunctuated sentences without ever showing any sign of shortness of breath. Yet they do not create the kind of tension in the air that many fast speakers do; their words actually roll quite pleasantly like water in a creek.

Their clinic is located in a nondescript commercial building, and the clinic waiting area is minimally decorated, with no frills whatsoever. A small side table that has a tray with clean cups and a glass jug of water shows consideration and the beauty of simplicity. After all, it is highly recommended by most practitioners for the patients to drink some water after treatments.

Joy had always been in the healthcare profession. In her work as a registered nurse in the intensive care unit, Joy saw not only how Western biomedicine saves lives, but also how it compromises with countless side effects. She was quick to realize that sometimes the side effects were so severe that it was the side effects that were putting patients into hospitals, not the illnesses. And she grew increasingly critical of the lack of preventive measures for some of the chronic conditions that she so often saw gradually become too severe to be reversed by medical treatments.

In the early 1980s, out of frustration toward Western biomedicine and to take a break from her high stress job, she decided to take a six-month sabbatical. She went to Taiwan to learn Mandarin Chinese and more about *taichi*, which she had already started to practice, and ended up staying in Taiwan for four years. During her stay, her encounters with traditional Chinese medicine were so frequent that she felt it was almost fate for her to study acupuncture. She noticed individuals who provided traditional healing to others, sometimes for fees but other times for free. A friend was interning with an acupuncturist who gave free services at local temples and community centers, and Joy finally decided to go along and observe. The acupuncturists greeted the patients, made diagnoses, and instructed the interns to administer acupuncture and suction cups at designated points. Sometimes there were tables, and sometimes the patients had to be treated in chairs, but nothing stopped the patients from coming.

The experience of observing the treatments got Joy interested, but not completely convinced. With her biomedical background (and a personal fear of needles, she admitted), she was still suspicious toward the effectiveness of traditional Chinese healing. She remembers one particular incident that brought her to the realization that really changed her perspective toward acupuncture. She had a nagging toothache for a week, and mentioned her discomfort to a friend. The friend offered to give her a treatment, with just one needle:

> He got me in the car, and he strapped me in and twisted, and in a few minutes, I felt like a numbing sensation around where my toothache was. He said, we'll keep the needle in for about twenty minutes. Then he took the needle off, and you know that numbing feeling . . . so that the toothache was much less by that time. So I was like hmmm this is quite interesting, it works, it works. So I was still not 100 percent convinced because . . . toothache means you got a tooth infection on the tooth canal . . . by that night [the pain] was almost gone . . . by the next morning it was gone completely. No toothache.

Growing up in a Chinese household, Joy had always known that the "nasty tasting concoctions" that her mother gave to her worked, but she had never had acupuncture before this. She still found a dentist the next day to check on her tooth, who told her that although the filling came off, the tooth had no inflammation at all. She was amazed:

> I said, if it is powerful enough to do THAT, and it's got three or four thousand years of continuous use, it must have some validity, and you know if it didn't work it would have died out by now. It wouldn't even last a few thousand years so that's when I truly started becoming more interested in acupuncture.

Joy then found that there were acupuncture schools in the Bay Area, so she applied and finally came home. However, even when she was studying in the acupuncture program, she was still undecided on whether she would completely abandon nursing. Then a health condition helped her make up her mind. During the second year of her acupuncture program, Joy was diagnosed with a thyroid condition. Her biomedical doctor recommended radioactive thyroid treatment, but Joy was wary that the radioactive therapy would cause too much damage to her thyroid glands. She decided it was time to put traditional Chinese medicine into use. Alongside her biomedical medication, she also supplemented with herbal formulae and acupuncture. As the dosage of her biomedical prescription slowly decreased, the TCM treatments helped her become stronger and healthier again. She was able to preserve the function of her thyroid, and also to restore her health enough to conceive a child. Her pregnancy was normal, and both she and the child have been healthy.

Joy used to teach at one of the TCM colleges, but stopped teaching when she got pregnant. She also worked in two clinics, and now cuts down to working only part-time in one clinic to be able to accommodate her child's schedule. The life of a working mother is never easy, which many of her patients must find themselves identifying with readily.

While Joy tells her story, Adam listens to his wife speak with attention and smiles. Unlike most California-trained practitioners in his generation, acupuncture was Adam's first career. He majored in music as an undergraduate, but could not see himself teaching music. After first toying with the idea of law school, he realized that his passion was in health and taking care of people. Having always had interest in herbal medicine and the long history of Chinese medicine, he took an introductory course in one of the TCM schools before he graduated from college, and by the time he received his bachelor's degree, he decided to enroll in the TCM program.

As if destiny had things all lined up for him, upon graduating from the TCM program, a Japanese friend from school had a connection with a new Japanese-style acupuncture school in town, which secured Adam a job immediately. He also had the opportunity of a clinical job, so he was an administrator-practitioner from the beginning. As the only Caucasian American administrator at the new school, he had a heavy dose of Japanese culture and Japanese-style acupuncture from the job. Adam also struggled with the notion that he might eventually turn into an administrator who only nominally has the title of an acupuncturist, but with no time to maintain clinical competency.

Having seen acupuncture practices beyond the Bay Area (as Joy had seen in Taiwan) and outside of the TCM paradigm (as Adam had seen in the Japanese acupuncture school and Japanese-style practitioners), Joy and Adam are very aware of the limitations of the training offered by the TCM schools in the Bay Area. For one, they believe that the TCM circle in the Bay Area is not as sophisticated about other practices of acupuncture or traditional Chinese medicine that they have encountered. Adam points out that many of the practitioners from Mainland China were herbalists by training, and Joy adds that some of her professors in the TCM school were MDs in China, who may have had training in TCM but were by no means specialists in the tradition. Adam compares the hands-on aspect of acupuncture with the doctors of osteopath in the United States:

> [With] needles there's a lot of skill of application of the needle, and also there's a lot of—it's also hands-on, which professionally is the lowest level. Every profession . . . health profession . . . where you touch people, that's actually lowest level, socially [and] culturally. Something I realize having an osteopath teacher; she said that in United States, osteopathy went out because it's low level to be touching people, which is funny in the age we live in. I think [the touching aspect is] actually getting more importance, because people need more touching. But realistically—traditionally for those people from China came here, where there's more herbalists 'cause it was a more practical approach when you had many people you were dealing with. There were issues of also the low status of people who actually do these hands-on things.

When I start to steer the discussion toward the relationship between traditional Chinese medicine and spirituality, the pair have much to say. Adam again references the Japanese perspective:

> If you look historically, [spirituality] wasn't in the medicine; it was just considered that medicine does have spiritual dimension, because it's serving health of others and it's very intimate with people. So in that sense there might be some spiritual practice to use, to kind of energize, because especially with Japanese, when you are touching people, it's like, how good is your touch? And your touch is affected by having a good spiritual practice. I mean most people believe that.

Adam then brings the Christian faith into the mix:

> You must have interviewed Chinese practitioners that are very Christian, right? They put Christian spirituality into their parts of Chinese medicine. The people I work with are exactly like that. They are very Christian and very into Chinese medicine, and there's been a lot of people like that.

Joy chimes in with an anecdote she personally encountered:

> I remember about this patient of mine. After I had been treating her for a while, she asked me whether I say a prayer when I put the needles in, or if I do some kind of incantation. (Adam comments, "Because the patient is Christian you see, they are very scared.") I was really taken back because no one has ever asked me that kind of question before. I said, no, I just read your pulse and find out your imbalance, and then I put the needles in according to what your condition is.

However, Joy also tells the patient that although she does not say a prayer herself, she thinks that prayers can be important to individuals who have spiritual beliefs. Then the patient shared something shocking—the patient's pastor told her that acupuncture is devil's work:

> As it turned out her pastor warned her to not go to acupuncture because it's like voodoo or something, the devils work and you never know what they are going to do to you, like witchcraft. I thought, wow, this is really intense. This is a woman who was having chemotherapy, who was so sick when she came to see me, and got so much better, and she is listening to her pastor, and she stopped coming for her treatments. Obviously my answer didn't satisfy her. She was still influenced by her pastor who didn't do a thing to help her recover.

Saddened by the pastor's defamation of TCM, and more so by the fact that her patient, who could have benefited significantly from the acupuncture treatment, heeded her pastor's persuasion, she says,

> Maybe he prayed for her, hopefully he did. I thought, wow, here are people that are in such positions of influence, who are so ignorant and they are influencing masses of people, so that they can't get the medical help they need because of some weird misunderstanding or fear. It's totally ignorant because obviously they don't understand anything to do with the medicine. They haven't read anything about the history of Chinese medicine and what it does. But they are giving these ideas to their congregations! I was completely taken aback and so I thought oh there are these thoughts circulating.

On the other hand, Adam asserts, some practitioners may be infusing too much of the "spiritual" into the medicine without enough validation:

> Chinese medicine is holistic medicine, which is very nice. It's pretty enlightening where you don't divide the body and mind and that's very important. It's very important to treat people as a whole person. But sometimes it seems to me like some of the other people at the school treat the extra-meridians for emotions, like they are stuck at this level, so we need to free that. I'm just not that convinced that they know what they are talking about. . . . Acupuncture is profoundly relaxing and people feel really good after it anyway.

Adam goes on to remind us that the non-separation between spiritual and physical should be basic understanding for practitioners of Chinese medicine:

> [Some practitioners] are not seeing [that] if you treat the physical side, you'll also treat the spiritual side, that they are not separate. That's day one of Chinese medicine. It's not separate. Spirituality as we conceive it in the West . . . is very non-physical isn't it? It's kind of divorced from the physical and that's a carry-through of our culture . . . how it's so separate.

To Joy, it is the "Spirituality in California," which she sees in her clinical encounters with patients as well:

> The spirituality in California is very different, and that's why sometimes when you treat patients, you may be treating them for a physical condition they have, then all of a sudden they burst into tears. Or they have a crisis, and it becomes spiritual for them in a sense, because somehow [the acupuncture treatment] unblocks something in their body, which made them able to experience or to go through whatever they needed to go through as part of their healing. It's not like I did anything special. I didn't look for that special unblocking point.

Even though she does not provide anything spiritual in her treatment, Joy understands that because of the non-separation between physical and other dimensions, her patients' needs beyond the physical are also met in the process:

> I remember once one of my patients said she had been having migraines for a long time before she came to have treatments with me. She said she felt like she was having an out-of-body experience while she was having a treatment, and after that day her migraines completely disappeared and they were completely gone. I said I didn't do anything special to facilitate that, all I did was treat her for what I felt like she needed to be treated, and whatever it was it just helped her to be able to break into that. So her own body allowed her to, because of the treatment, be able to transcend or be able to open up or whatever it is. I'm not a psychologist, so I can't really do counseling.

She explains how, without doing anything beyond treating the physical, she is able to heal her patients' concerns that are beyond physical:

> As people say, acupuncture can do some much, not just for the physical but mental and emotional, because it opens up the meridians, and allows the flow of energy. Things that are locked up become revealed. Some people say it helps their creativity, (Adam: Yeah.) because it gets things moving . . . [after some unblocking] they're able to tap into that creativity side and intuition. It's not like it's a special fantastic miracle point.

It is interesting that as Joy starts to touch upon what is almost a threshold to "spiritual," Adam points to the "cultural" sources of concepts such as *gui*, or ghost:

> Some of these old Chinese practitioners who do [acupuncture to exorcise] the ghosts and things like that—that's very cultural right? That's not really Chinese medicine per se. If you read like Unschuld's thing, he's saying that's cultural . . . Chinese medicine with a small c, because it's generic to China and a basic culture. But it's not Chinese medicine of Neijing and Nanjing, the original classics.

Joy counters his assessment of the differentiations between spiritual and cultural, and classic versus modern:

> I remember there's some old Chinese medical text talked about the causes of disease—cold and heat, and the last one was *gui*, which is ghost. Now of course some modern people have taken that interpreted as pathogens because back then they could not explain.

Adam quickly snaps back:

> But even that, *gui*. There is actually an acupuncture treatment . . . it's even more recent; it's like a later part of acupuncture that did more of that, in Qing and Ming. If you read *Shanghan Lun*, there's nothing about *gui*, it's all about *shanghan* (typhoid, or literally, cold damage). It's a part of the culture but actually there's an illusion that it goes way back, when in fact it only goes back maybe a few hundred years.
> [Things like possession] go way way back, but Chinese medicine . . . if you read the *Neijing*, where do they talk about *gui* in there? They don't talk about it anywhere. So they were consciously talking about nature and living with the rhythm of nature. They had *daoyin*(??) and things like that to be more specific than nature but they were concerned with that.

Joy and I joined forces in reminding him that there must be different variants in medical thought through the long history of Chinese medicine. Daoist texts, for example, have a long history of talking about the human body with concepts of gods and spirits residing in different inner organs and body parts. Translation and interpretation issues should also be considered, says Joy:

> The other thing is ghosts points . . . the Chinese characters of the point names. There are so many meanings for them. Sometimes you have to look at what are the possibilities for the interpretation rather than the one word. So I think that's the problem with translations sometimes, because when you translate something and especially some of these old classical texts, they could go back and forth about this one character of what it means and they could hold seminars about the possibilities. And those books are all written about these bamboo strips and at some point the strips get all mixed up and a strip is missing. Then for centu-

ries later you are trying to piece things together and make sense of them and still have different interpretations.

Without a conclusive or decisive position on either side of the discussion, it soon became apparent that perhaps discussions such as this are typical of their daily interactions. Adam hinted at the conflict of interests between the spiritual implications in medicine and the mainstream medical care system:

> Holistic medicine leads itself to people with spiritual inclinations, because it's holistic and you think of treating the whole person. It should be the concern of all medicine, really. Medicine [in general] does have spiritual implications at some point. There's a lot of denial of it in mainstream medical care because it may get in the way of a profit here and there.

VERA[2] (LICENSED ACUPUNCTURIST IN PRIVATE PRACTICE; PROFESSOR AND CLINIC SUPERVISOR AT TCM SCHOOL; HEAD OF LABORATORY AT TCM SCHOOL CLINIC)

We met Vera in Chapter 3, where I observed her work at a TCM school's ear clinic. Vera also allowed me to interview her in her clinic. Her private practice in the city of San Francisco is inside an old house that she shares with a few other practitioners. The weathered wooden floor, small doors, and narrow hallways exude the kind of charm that only comes with time and constant human usage. Vera's office has a unique lived-in feel, more like a tenured professor's office than a clinician's workspace: piles of papers and books cover the desk, and the walls are decorated by posters and photos of people practicing martial arts. With her long golden hair casually pulled back into a low ponytail, Vera comes across as down-to-earth, practical, and very approachable.

She points to one poster that shows a young Caucasian woman doing a high kick, "See, that is me thirty years ago. They thought it was interesting to see a blond girl doing martial arts, so they put on me the poster."

Vera very quickly got into her life story leading to where she is now, a practitioner of traditional Chinese medicine who also teaches in a local TCM school. She came from a biology background and worked as a medical technologist in the biotech industry for a few years.

"I got disinterested in Western medical degrees and research when I worked in biotech in the early 70s with people who were doing research in medicine who were trying to sell products." Vera further recalls:

> The products that I was working on were instruments that were for medical labs, so that you can do blood sugar tests in the hospital or you can do all kinds of things. And what I learned is that people would lie and alter data so that their product could get out on the market. I once worked with doctors, women doctors mostly, who would say, I left

teaching at the medical school research because my colleagues were lying about their data so the drug companies would hire them.

Disappointed by the capitalist orientation of a major biotechnological corporation, she left New York for San Francisco, where she started to pursue a healthier lifestyle and a career as a biomedical physician. Vera's new life in San Francisco presented her with unexpected trajectories. Some of her old friends from college just returned from Japan after learning a form of martial art called *shintaido* 新体道, and wanted to start a school in San Francisco. They found a place to live together. And when their *sensei* arrived from Japan a few months later, Vera also helped them with founding a non-profit organization to teach *shintaido*. To Vera, her interest in martial art was not in the fighting or competition, but in how it promotes peace.

"*Shintaido* means 'New Body Way,' and it was founded to take a healthy body . . . much like *taichi* or *qigong* . . . and building up your body's *qi*, and then using it to heal things rather than to fight." Vera explains why she was attracted to this particular type of martial art. "You take the energy of somebody who's trying to come at you and attack, and you turn them around and you go into a new vector where both of you will become better."

A form that originated from karate, *shintaido* was created in 1965 by Hiroyuki Aoki, who was an actor, painter, and karate master, to explore "the unknown world which begins at the end of our psychological strength."[3] Aoki blends traditional Japanese martial techniques with wisdoms of Buddhist meditation and traditional Chinese medicine to "infuse the rigorous martial arts tradition with creative expression."[4] Although the official rhetoric of Shintaido of America no longer mentions Christian influences, early students like Vera remember how the martial art embraced the kind of universal, humanistic compassion exemplified by Christian civil rights leaders like Martin Luther King, Jr.

Vera's practice of *shintaido* and enthusiasm for the martial art took her to Japan in 1979, where she met *shintaido* teachers who also practiced Japanese acupuncture. She was so fascinated that she would have studied in Japan with them, but the acupuncture program in Japan required that she read and write Japanese fluently. She returned to San Francisco to attend a Japanese *shiatsu* school, but decided that she wanted to attend a program with more "medicine," even if she was not going to go to a biomedical school.

The practice and cultivation with *shintaido* and the revelations Vera gained from it may also have directly influenced her approach to the practice of traditional Chinese medicine:

> Chinese medicine was appealing to me because there is a rigor that you have to learn about the truth, about being truthful, about what you are feeling about your patients. And it's not just in your mind that you are

feeling that this person is anxious and therefore we are going to choose this point for anxiety.

She talks more about what she means by "being truthful":

So in order to do a good job giving acupuncture treatments, case by case, you are truly feeling the pulse, looking at the tongue, and really, really just looking at the body in front of you and knowing what's supposed to happen. And not being skewed by what they tell you or what you already thought about, or what was true last week. You see this today and this is the treatment. You feel what level of *qi* this person has in their body, and you know what you are supposed to do to balance that body. It's very pure and very nice. It's a very together system, that is, if you apply the template of pure Chinese medicine each time correctly, then you always get the truth about the patient.

With this truthful and humanitarian spirit, Vera not only runs her own practice and teaches at a TCM school, she also volunteers. When she arrived at San Francisco thirty years ago, she visited a free clinic with a friend. The clinic offered free services for a wide range of conditions, and Vera got especially interested in their free services for the people with substance abuse issues. She started with volunteering her service at their clinic laboratory, and thirty years later, she still volunteers there as the director of their small laboratory. When she later became an acupuncturist, she also provided free acupuncture treatments. As a supervising faculty member at the TCM school, she also has some of her student interns work at the free clinic.

Vera sees the problem of biomedicine not so much in the medicine itself, but in the business or market orientation of the medicine, particularly the domination of health insurance companies over the medical field:

[Biomedical physicians] have gone away from their physical exams skills and their using of lab tests. That's OK. Actually, the problem they are having now is letting the health insurance companies to just take over. They are allowing non-medical, non-physician decisions to direct how they proceed with treatment or diagnosing people. And they are getting into big trouble with that. And in a way, who cares, because if you have money you can always bypass that system and hire a doctor who will just really take care of you, spend time looking at you. But if you are just a poor person with a [standard health insurance] plan, you are only going to get that kind of way. Not good. Not good at all.

And acupuncturists also inevitably participate in the reality of being under the control or at least the influence of health insurance companies. Current insurance policies have very limited coverage for acupuncture treatments, if acupuncture is covered at all. Acupuncturists who petition on behalf of their patients essentially volunteer their time during the process of letter writing and negotiations, with their requests often not being granted. On the other hand, biomedical physicians are paid for their time to provide similar medical reports. Vera expresses genuine concerns when she explains the challenges that she and her fellow colleagues face on a regular basis, "It's very hard to make a living like this in an expensive city like ours."

DR. YUAN (LICENSED ACUPUNCTURIST IN PRIVATE PRACTICE; PROFESSOR AND CLINIC SUPERVISOR AT A TCM SCHOOL)[5]

A talented acupuncturist who specializes in cardiology, Dr. Yuan became the chief physician at a prestigious hospital in Shanghai when he was only thirty years old. In 1997, his wife, a genetic scientist, found a job in the Bay Area. The couple, with their toddler son in tow, immigrated to America. It was a time when the near-complete Human Genome Project was the talk of the world, and the field of genetic science was on the rise. Mrs. Yuan loved her job. She found her job both challenging and rewarding, and for the first few years they were in the Bay Area, she was the main breadwinner of the family.

In those early years, Dr. Yuan's Chinese friends and students often wondered how he managed emotionally. After all, he gave up his highly respected position and promising career in China to support his wife's career. Here he found himself struggling with the English language and fast becoming the homemaker of the family, cooking meals and caring for their young son while his wife worked overtime. He was also teaching at the local TCM schools part-time for the meager $25 hourly wage. Worst of all, he wanted to practice clinically, but found himself, both financially and mentally, completely unprepared to set up and operate a private practice.

In China, Dr. Yuan knew he was a skillful doctor; all he had to focus on was to treat the patients who came in, and they flowed in nonstop. It never occurred to him that he would one day have to worry about money or how to run a business. He was surprised and frustrated by the tedious errands and social networking unavoidable in a small private practice in America. When he first started his own business, he often sat in the tiny yet empty clinic wondering how he could get the patients to come to him. Finally he gathered up enough courage to visit all the other businesses in the complex and introduce himself to them. That was the first time Dr. Yuan had to make himself socialize with others rather than having others come to him. Highly respected by his students at the TCM school, Dr. Yuan also gets referrals from his students and through word of mouth in the grapevine of the local Chinese community.

After years of running a relatively successful clinic, Dr. Yuan still resists the concept of running a business:

> I never had to think about business. People who study medicine graduate and get sent to places that need them, and you just do your doctoring. The relationship between the doctor and the patient is strictly a clinical relationship, and you do not worry about other aspects of the patients. Business and money had very little to do with me. The rest is whether your [clinical] skills meet the demands, otherwise you don't have to worry. Here it is completely different. Here I have to depend on myself. I have to be in charge of money and business. It's completely different.

The business operation was not the only aspect of the American medical framework that Dr. Yuan had to adjust to. In the hospital he worked in, TCM was fully integrated with biomedicine. As a TCM cardiologist, he had full access to biomedical tools and exams for diagnosis, and used acupuncture and Chinese herbs alongside pharmaceutical medication. He also worked alongside biomedical surgeons to provide pre-surgery and post-surgery care. Without biomedical credentials in the United States, Dr. Yuan finds himself limited—rather than directly ordering exams and prescribing pharmaceutical medications that he knows would be more effective and appropriate for the conditions of some of his patients, he can now merely make suggestions for the patients to urge their biomedical physicians to take action. "Sometimes I know something is very wrong, but the patient's specialist may not agree with me," says Dr. Yuan, with a little frustration in his voice, "I do what I can. Some patients trust me enough to ask for my opinion, but whatever I say can only be for their reference if their conditions require more help than acupuncture and herbs."

In his simple clinic with two small treatment rooms, Dr. Yuan currently runs a general practice. He is always confident clinically, especially with Chinese patients. Rigorous in keeping up with the newest clinical findings from Mainland China, Dr. Yuan is still deeply connected to the pulses of the source of medical knowledge that he once participated in and was forced to "leave behind."

Closely associated with his fear of losing touch with the authentic source of knowledge on TCM is his perception of an unbridgeable language gap. Even after a decade of practice in the Bay Area, he believes that the language barrier still creates clinical difficulties:

> Language is a big problem. [Traditional] Chinese medicine is not easy to explain because it is very abstract. If I want to be precise about what diseases and etiologies are involved, that's hard to explain. In Chinese I can do much better, but in English I find it difficult. What causes the illness? How are the symptoms going to progress? What are the etiologies? What good will this treatment do for you? These are more difficult. Biomedical etiologies also get complicated, but then the Western doctors don't usually explain very clearly [to their patients] either.

Amidst our conversation, a Caucasian American man enters the clinic to make an inquiry. The clearly distraught man explains that his wife has been diagnosed with cancer, and he wants to know if acupuncture could help her at all. Dr. Yuan listens patiently, and explains to the man the benefits and limitations of acupuncture treatments for cancer patients. His English is slow but clear, and within minutes the man is calmed significantly. Finally, Dr. Yuan hands the man a business card, and encourages him to call back for an appointment if his wife is interested. The man leaves with an obviously lighter spirit.

As the man closes the clinic door after him and while Dr. Yuan's waving hand is still in midair, I turn to him and say, "I think you are being too harsh on yourself about English, Dr. Yuan."

"You know the old Chinese saying," Dr. Yuan says, almost sheepishly. "There is no end to learning (*xuewu zhijing* 學無止境). And I honestly don't think my English is any good. I still feel so embarrassed every time I have to speak it."

I look past his shoulders, at the carrying case of the electrocardiography machine that he was showing me before the man came in. He only uses it occasionally now to help monitor the few patients who have heart problems. I ask him if he misses those days when he had much more biomedical authority and resources to practice a more integrated medicine. "Not really," he explains. "During the Cultural Revolution [in China], sometimes doctors had nothing but a few needles they made from the spokes of bike wheels, and they still had to somehow help their patients. We are lucky that we are not in that situation now, and that patients have their Western doctors to go to. It's just a different world." He sighs. "It's just a very different world."

RECAP: PRACTICING BETTER MEDICINE

While also emphasizing the importance of mastering biomedical knowledge, this group of TCM practitioners differs from the previous group by positioning themselves decidedly outside of biomedicine. The dissatisfaction these practitioners feel toward biomedicine, for varying reasons, motivates them to offer alternative healing to patients, and they do not work directly with biomedical physicians on a regular basis. They may have referral relationships with some biomedical physicians, whereby from word of mouth the physicians refer their patients to these practitioners for acupuncture treatments. There are limited actual interactions or intellectual exchanges between practitioners and the physicians who refer patients to them. Very often, the communication is through the patients rather than between the practitioners and the physicians directly.

Whereas the complementary practitioners who work within biomedical institutions have access to the social and financial resources as part of the biomedical cohort, the alternative practitioners do not seem to have the kind of close personal relationships that lend them biomedical endorsement. On the other hand, these alternative practitioners, who have previously worked within or in close proximity to the biomedical system—Joy as a nurse, Vera as a pharmaceutical technician, and Dr. Yuan as a PRC-TCM cardiologist—are familiar with biomedical diagnoses, procedures, and laboratory tests. Most importantly, such familiarity allows them to distinguish themselves from what they believe are shortcomings of biomedical system, and provide what they believe are proper treatments to the patients. In this type of distinction, power and authority comes from identifying problems in biomedicine, and providing TCM solutions to those problems.

Without the strong financial backing of biomedical institutions to conduct evidence-based research, the patients' subjective experiences in the clinic become an important basis for assessing the clinical efficacy of TCM treatments performed by alternative mode practitioners. Interestingly, perhaps influenced by their biomedical training or their conception of healing practices based on the "scientific" biomedical model, the practitioners in this group acknowledge incorporating bodily and qi cultivation in their practices, but do not necessarily see themselves needing to utilize other spiritually related resources.

NOTES

1. Personal interview, May 12, 2008. The interview was conducted in English.
2. Personal interview, May 6, 2008. The interview was conducted in English.
3. "What is Shintaido: The Shintaido Story," on Shintaido of America website, http://www.shintaido.org/docs/history.htm (accessed May 27, 2012).
4. Ibid.
5. Personal interview, September 20, 2008. Interview was conducted entirely in Mandarin Chinese, and quotes were translated into English by the author.

SEVEN
Creating a Space for Psychic Healing

There is no question that a significant number of practitioners were attracted to TCM for its being holistic and supposedly inclusive of the spiritual dimension of health. Most of the practitioners interested in spiritual healing explore the theoretical and technical aspects of tapping into healing patients holistically. However, a very small percentage of the practitioners I interviewed possess very strong psychic abilities that they incorporate into their clinical practices. In this chapter, the psychic practitioners share their challenges as people who are aware of the negative perceptions of psychics as mentally unstable and deceptive, and found who TCM a medical profession that allows them to put their rare gifts into proper therapeutic use.

TARA (LICENSED ACUPUNCTURIST IN PRIVATE PRACTICE; FERTILITY SPECIALIZATION)[1]

The colors of the clinic interior are soft and soothing, and the ceilings are covered by cascading waves of soft fabric. The lighting is intentionally dim, and images of bodhisattvas grace the walls. Amidst the softly appealing decor, Tara and her friend who helps out at the clinic enliven the atmosphere with their humorous chitchat and laughter. A deck of intricately illustrated inspirational cards on the reception counter catches my attention. "Pick a card," prompts Tara. "See what you get. My patients always get excited by what the cards have to say to them."

Tara has porcelain skin, hair in impressive spiral curls, and a silvery voice. Previously a graphic designer, she obviously brought her sense of aesthetics into her clinic and her person. Always interested in natural medicine, she spent many years contemplating going to medical school, but the idea of spending about ten years to get through science prerequisites, medical school, and residency seemed far-fetched. In 1991 she moved from New York to California, and a career crisis prompted her to consider medical school again. Having been previously treated by an acupuncturist in Boston and impressed by the efficacy of the treatments, Tara had a revelation:

> One day I was sitting in my living room. I lived in Sacramento at the time and it was like a light bulb went off in my head, and I thought, I could study acupuncture! Oh that's beautiful! It's a blending of science, and a blending of a natural medicine that I liked because they used herbs. And it's not drug-related. And it felt like the right thing to do.

After training in a TCM school in the Bay Area and attaining a state acupuncture license, Tara first practiced in San Francisco. Gradually, she started to focus her practice more and more on fertility treatments, and moved out of San Francisco to several different locations in the northern part of the Bay Area until finally settling down in Marin County.

Fertility has been an emerging specialty among acupuncturists in the Bay Area in the recent decade. While there had been Western clinical studies on efficacy of acupuncture in several aspects of reproductive health published since the early 1990s, the breakthrough evidence-based study was a German paper published in 2001 on the significant increase in the success rate when patients undergoing in vitro fertility treatment also receive acupuncture treatments.[2] Many biomedical fertility clinics started to actively refer their patients to acupuncturists, and more acupuncturists who saw the potential of the niche started to specialize in fertility treatments, often establishing working relationships with biomedical fertility clinics.

Tara is a fellow of the American Board of Oriental Reproductive Medicine (ABORM), a small national specialty board with certified practitioners in twenty-six states in the United States and British Columbia in Canada. Among all 113 certified practitioners listed on ABORM's website, 48 of them practice in California, and 26 (23 percent, or almost a quarter) practice in the San Francisco Bay Area.[3] ABORM certifies licensed acupuncturists by its own examination, and offers continuing education units specifically in fertility-related topics.[4] Acupuncturists are not legally required by the state of California to be certified by ABORM to claim a specialty in fertility; out of the four practitioners I interviewed whose clinics exclusively treat fertility clients, only Tara is certified by ABORM. However, all four practitioners have booming businesses, and one of them told me that if I ever consider becoming an acupuncturist myself, I should remember that fertility is where the money goes.

While high demand for fertility treatments has brought economic fortunes to the practitioners, some of those who seek these treatments are emotionally high-maintenance clients. Tara characterizes her clients:

> I don't get the relaxed person in here who is suffering from infertility; I get the type-A personality that's burning the candle at both ends. . . . [W]hen you are that tightly wound you are tuned out to that aspect of your life. A lot of people are tuned out of their bodies, and they are not as aware of their bodies, so they have to relearn all these things when they come.

Her patients often realize that they see her for not only the physical treatment but also psychological therapy:

> Fertility is highly charged and you have to deal with the emotional aspect of fertility. [The patient is] not just a sitting uterus to me, [she is] a person who has thoughts and feelings and is struggling. It's a huge struggle for a couple, a woman facing fertility issues, huge because it's at the core of femininity. So we do have lots of emotional discussions. But I will say most of the people, the majority of the people, that I see are healthy and they are willing to examine themselves.

Although both men and women can have fertility problems, Tara observes something interesting in her practice:

> The women all take charge, but even though sometimes there's nothing wrong with [the woman] clinically [she tests] fine, all [her] lab tests are normal, [her] uterus is fine, [her] ovaries, [her] fallopian tubes . . . there's nothing wrong with [her], but it's the husband's sperms that are terrible, [the women] are still the ones who are coming to see me regularly.

Occasionally she gets calls asking if she could perform the impossible:

> Then I get [women] call me at like [age] fifty-one, can I have a baby? Can you help me have a baby? I have a young boyfriend, [and] he would like to have children. Can you help me get pregnant? Are you having regular menstrual cycles? Oh no, no, no that stopped a year ago. I'm like, I can't do nothing for you. I'm not a miracle worker.

The patients can get too psychologically demanding and morally taxing for her to handle:

> One woman, I know this is going to sound out there, but when she left I just talked to her soul and told her I don't want to see you anymore, you need to see someone else and she cancelled her next appointment and I never saw her again.
>
> She had terminated a pregnancy that was a viable pregnancy at like six months. So this was a baby that was kicking and moving within her, and because she was having problems with her husband and she couldn't make the decision in the first trimester to terminate the pregnancy . . . she had to pay someone to do this because it's illegal to do . . . she paid somebody to terminate a healthy baby. And she was coming to me to get her pregnant again. And she was forty-four, and it was a year later; her body was starting to go into menopause. I decided I didn't feel right helping somebody like that because I never wanted to

be responsible. If I helped her get pregnant and she terminated that pregnancy too? So I chose, I didn't want to take her on.

Tara not only relies on her intuition to turn away morally problematic clients, she also has ways to energetically protect herself. She explains that she would first energetically expand her senses to where she feels an invisible yet tangible limit, and then pull back toward her physical body to create a bubble that shields her from things "not of her." The bubble is invisible to others, but in her visualization, the bubble is transparent with a rainbow-colored glare on the outside. This bubble creates an energetic separation between her and others, and protects her from the emotional, psychological, and psychical influences of her clients.

As I converse more with Tara, it becomes clear that she has an unconventional practice that, besides utilizing counseling and some telepathic communication, also incorporates diagnosis strategies that are far from the standard TCM school knowledge. Instead of checking the patient's pulse for conditions of the meridians, Tara uses a dowsing rod. She first studied with an acupuncturist who uses the dowsing rod to check whether the herbal formulae he prescribes to the patients are energetically suitable. A light bulb went off in Tara's head, and she tried using the dowsing rod to check the conditions of the patients' meridians directly. She enters the energy field of the patient with her dowsing rod, and the dowsing rod serves as a physical and visible pointer:

> If I want to I can go in [to your energy field] and I can see what your IQ is. It's called an energetic IQ, not your mental IQ, but your energetic IQ, which means the way that you're vibrating. Are you vibrating the way that you should be? There's a frequency that you should vibrate at when you're in the healthiest energetic form, and if you're not you have like what I call attachments. And attachments are things that happen with other people, because other people affect your energy field depending on how you let them come in. So you can check that. You can work on clearing those out. You can check and see how people's conditions are by the [dowsing rod's] spinning, how they are doing.

Tara uses nontraditional strategies to assist her in her interactions with the patients and in diagnoses and to make her treatment plans. On the other hand, her actual treatment strategies are quite standard: acupuncture in the appropriate points on the affected meridians and herbal formulae that she prescribes and hand-crafts from the "scientifically powdered herbs" (*kexue zhongyao* 科學中藥) into easy-to-consume capsules.

Creative integration of strategies from various sources into the acknowledged scope of practice for acupuncture (by the state license) is common among practitioners I talked to. Other practitioners are trained in several systems of complementary and alternative healing, and incorporate them all into their clinical practices. The next practitioner, Charles, is one example: he practices as a chiropractor, acupuncturist, and secretly as a psychic as well.

CHARLES (LICENSED CHIROPRACTOR AND LICENSED ACUPUNCTURIST IN PRIVATE PRACTICE; PSYCHIC)[5]

I sip from a cup of iced oolong tea at Charles's dining table while he leaves to answer the door. It is a friend of his wife, a lady speaking in Mandarin Chinese. Charles responds to her in Mandarin as well, "*Ta xianzai buzai jia* (she is not home right now)," with the imprecise tonality common in people who learn to speak the language later in their lives. *The pronunciation is clear and completely comprehensible though*, I catch myself musing inside my head.

Charles's wife is a Chinese immigrant, a beautiful, sweet woman, who appears to be fifteen to twenty years younger than he. When I show up at their house for the appointment, Charles has forgotten about it and his wife opens the door for me. She speaks to me in fluent English with a noticeable Chinese accent, quite parallel to the way Charles, a Caucasian American, speaks Chinese. Their house in a suburb of the Bay Area is new and spacious, with hints of Chinese around the house—a decoration here, a tea pot there—but from the outside it is just like other homes in the California suburb. Charles runs his medical practice in the basement of the house, a mixture of chiropractic and acupuncture, where he currently only takes male patients. Charles explains his unusual preference:

> Back in the eighties, we were able to use some chiropractic maneuvers that involve insertion of fingers and sometimes hand into the body. They were extremely effective and patients didn't have issues with them. Then some women patients started to sue for sexual harassment. Some of them came in looking to sue . . . you didn't even have to have done anything. The chiropractic programs no longer teach certain maneuvers now; it's really too bad for patients who could have benefited from them. And now I don't see female patients at all, to keep out of trouble.

A chiropractor for almost thirty years and an acupuncturist for almost twenty years, Charles teaches in both practices. There is no doubt that he is an experienced practitioner in both, but the way he talks about his combined practice makes little distinction between the two despite their different theoretical frameworks. Perhaps the distinctions do not matter so much for Charles, because he has a secret that none of his patients know: as soon as they walk into his door, he already knows what their illnesses or injuries are. More explicitly, Charles is a closeted psychic who diagnoses with his extrasensory ability, then uses chiropractic and acupuncture to treat the patients. He hides his psychic ability from his patients, often having to pretend that he reads their medical charts and checks their pulses before coming to conclusions:

> I ask them to bring in their charts and I take my time reading the lab results, and nod and pretend to pay very good attention to what they complain about. Actually, I already know what their problems are when they walk in. In all these years I have been practicing, I have only been "off" once. My antenna must have been disturbed that day. But that's about one in three thousand of a chance to make a mistake.

When Charles talks about his psychic abilities, he expresses both pride and caution. He worries that his voice can possibly be recognized by others in the medical professions or his patients, and requests that part of the interview be off the recording. On the other hand, he spends hours telling me the story of his life and the eventful path he took to become who he is today. He is obviously very aware of people's negative perceptions of psychic healers as charlatans, and shows his attempt to legitimize his medical practices by his extensive training, clinical and teaching experiences in chiropractic and traditional Chinese medicine. Things that other Caucasian American practitioners do to bolster their professional credibility—multiple certificates in specialty training, clinical internship in China, and teaching in the local TCM schools—Charles has done them all, and lists them in a lengthy curriculum vitae that is available on the internet.

When Charles was a teen, he went through a surgery that almost took his life. The near-death experience not only impacted him emotionally, it also left him with a side effect—he became a psychic. He started to have visions that predicted future events, and realized that he could locate his friends if they allowed him to find them (like a human version of satellite tracking system, if you will).

A rebellious youth who lived in the revolutionary 1970s, Charles dropped out of college to experience life. With his favorite poetry collection in his backpack and a five-dollar bill in his pocket, Charles found himself collecting seaweed along the coast of California to sell to the toothpaste manufacturers (apparently seaweed is a main ingredient in toothpastes). The non-contract labor made him just enough money for food, but allowed for total freedom to wander and roam, both physically and intellectually.

Then came another fateful day. Charles was taking a break from the day's work, and decided to nap on the lawn in a public parking lot by the seashore. A truck drove into the parking lot, and when the truck driver saw that all the parking spots were taken, he decided to park his truck on the lawn. The driver must had not seen or expected Charles there, because the truck's wheels ran right over Charles's knees—both knees. Worse yet, when Charles woke up from the sudden pain and screamed, the truck driver panicked and backed up the truck, running the wheels over Charles's knees *a second time*. The truck driver and shocked bystanders found Charles with his knees bending backward, and rushed him to the nearest medical clinic.

When the doctor saw the state of Charles's injuries, he recommended immediate surgery, but Charles had a different idea. He pulled his pants pockets inside out and said to the doctor, "I have no health insurance, and only have $50 on me. Do you really want to perform a surgery and provide after-surgery care that I cannot possibly pay you back for?" This was a small Seventh Day Adventist hospital that had only two doctors and nine beds. He would have potentially taken up more than ten percent of their total beds. Instead, he struck a deal with the doctor. He would borrow full braces and crutches from the doctor, and would try to heal himself. He promised to return the braces and crutches and, upon returning them, pay the doctor $50 as rental fee. If he didn't walk into the clinic by himself in a month's time, he would then submit himself to the doctor and undergo operation.

Charles did not have any confidence in what he was doing, but allowed his intuition to lead him to what he felt was the right thing to do. The full braces on both legs made it hard for Charles to get up by himself, but with some help he got up and got himself out of the hospital. He hitchhiked and two Native American women picked him up, brought him home with them to a teepee in the forest, and treated his knees with herbs from the forest, mashed and mixed into a paste. The women taught him how to find and use the herbs, and he continued to treat himself after three days of staying with them. In a month's time he walked into the clinic, and the doctor looked at him as if he were a ghost. He asked for braces that could bend at the knees, and eventually recovered fully.

The knee-injury incident brought Charles to two things that became pivotal in his life: esoteric spirituality and healing. Charles currently self-identifies as a freemason and a Gnostic, and frequently participates in Native American ceremonies and rituals. He makes it clear that spiritual experiences were, and still are, fundamental to the development and evolution of his psychic abilities.

Chiropractic also came to Charles with a traumatic entrance. After a few years of nomadic life along the California coast, he settled down in a small town with a girlfriend. He found a job, and life became more grounded. At the same time, he realized that he started to lose weight rapidly no matter how much he was eating, and ingestion of the smallest trace of fat made him gravely ill. Some friends suggested that he visit a chiropractor, who then diagnosed Charles with an obstructed bile duct, a condition that normally requires surgery to correct. The chiropractor performed some maneuvers on Charles, and after only one treatment, not only was Charles's bile duct unblocked, he somehow gained a new vision of the world:

124   Chapter 7

> I always knew that I didn't see colors as brightly as other people do, but it was not really that much of an issue. Then after that one treatment, I walked out of the clinic and the sky was in a blue so vivid that I have never seen a blue like that before. All the colors of the world suddenly came alive.

Charles almost immediately decided that he would pursue a career in chiropractic. Motivated by the transformational experience, he went back to school to complete the required prerequisite courses to apply to a chiropractic program. He made it into the chiropractic school with flying colors, but within two months, the school closed down. Determined to be trained, he and his friends took matters into their own hands. They bought old laboratory and clinic equipment from another school, and hired practicing local chiropractors to teach courses. Soon after, a major educational institution bought the school Charles and his friends started, which then became one of the leading chiropractic schools in California.

Interestingly, Charles does not specify another traumatic event that may have led him to traditional Chinese medicine. Deducing from his descriptions of the climates in the chiropractic profession, perhaps the frequent lawsuits and the fast diminishing list of "acceptable" maneuvers in chiropractic medicine made it necessary for him to acquire additional healing tools. Or perhaps an acupuncture license has gradually become a more competitive credential for the healthcare marketplace. Charles has created a legally legitimate and culturally accepted space for him to heal, although the psychic ability that he predominantly relies on to diagnose is not revealed to the patients.

DR. ZHANG (NON-LICENSED TCM HEALER, PSYCHIC)[6]

Through a small side entrance of a house, Dr. Zhang leads me through a garage, two flights of outdoor stairs, and into a small hidden studio that must have once been a storage space. The front part of the studio has barely enough room for a queen mattress, which serves also as the seating for a cramped computer desk against the wall, and the waiting area for visitors. There is a small kitchen on the side, within which Dr. Zhang somehow manages to fit a massage bed. She pulls a curtain to hide the kitchen stove and sink, but the smell of Chinese cooking and herbs fills the space.

A gaunt woman in her late forties, Dr. Zhang is very stern, and almost never smiles. She insists on being addressed as "Doctor," although she admits that she has no medical credentials of any kind in the United States or in her homeland China. In the nearby Yiguandao (一貫道)[7] temple where I met her, she volunteers in the free massage clinic, and designs recipes of nourishing soups and healing tonics for the temple kitchen, which provides free meals for members and visitors. Her Toisan[8] style recipes are popular among the Cantonese temple goers; she would sometimes prepare and sell packages of dry herbs and beans for stews. She is not a religious member of the temple, but the temple members know her as "the doctor at the temple." A few of the temple members schedule private, paid treatment sessions with her, either in the back room of the temple or at her house. Her regular income comes from her clinic hours at a local Chinese herb shop, three times a week.

Dr. Zhang came from the Guangdong province in China, and her father, a school principle, was an old-fashioned Confucian scholar. "My father was very proud of my older sister, because she was good at school," she reminiscent with a tone of grudge, "but you know how damaging the old feudal system could be to women! They lock women up at home and make them stupid!" Perhaps to prove her father wrong, Dr. Zhang took an unconventional path. Self-educated to become a healer, she remains unmarried, and uses some methods that her Confucian father would never approve of—psychic healing that involves spirits and ghosts that Confucius said "to never discuss," and manual techniques that requires touching patients, which would be considered by old Confucians to be improper especially if the patient is of the opposite sex.

In 1995, she started learning medical *qigong* from a master in the Shandong province, whose name she conveniently "forgets." This travelling master from the North regularly visited the Guangdong province in the South, where Dr. Zhang lived. She told her master that she not only wanted to heal with *qigong*, but she also wanted to be able to diagnose and heal at a distance. The master gave her some tips, "and I studied all the TCM books that I could find, and incorporated my life experiences," she shares with pride.

> I was able to do remote diagnosis and healing very soon after. If you understand the important principles and know how to apply theories in real life, even without a lot of clinical experience, you can still practice very effectively.

She then opened a private clinic with a partner, from whom she also learned many of the manual techniques that she uses. Through experimentation, she also developed some of her own manual techniques. Dr. Zhang is praised by some of her patients for her ability to manually adjust and align the spine and shoulder blades. During my visit, she happened to have a patient who wanted some adjustment in her slightly hunched upper back. With the patient lying face down on the massage bed, Dr. Zhang makes a fist with her right hand to hammer on the back of her patient. The fist on the flesh makes a dull "thump thump thump" sound. She hammers cautiously and consistently, like a blacksmith hammering on a piece of molten iron. With her fist still moving, she suddenly turns to ask, "Do you smell chives?"

"Chives? You mean if your neighbors are cooking chives?" I replied, taken by surprise.

"No, her back. You see this hump? When I hammer on it, it releases the smell of chives," she frowns. "You don't smell it? It's very strong. Sometimes when we eat food that we can't properly digest, the essence of food gets stored in different parts of our body, and we become congested." She pats the patient lightly on the shoulder to signal that she is talking to the patient, "This means your body is not efficient in digesting chives, so you shouldn't eat too much of it."

"So if you were able to release all the chive essence from the hump, the hump would go away?" I ask. This is an interesting theory—when digested food is improperly stored by the body, we can actually have a single food item, stored away in the body, that causes deformation.

"Oh yes," Dr. Zhang answers with no hesitation, and goes on to explain,

> Modern people consume too much cold food and do not dress warm enough, so most people are actually too cold (*han* 寒) to be healthy. A cold body is too weak to function properly, and on top of that, people eat foods that are difficult to digest or plain unhealthy for the body. A healthy body should digest food, transform food into essence (*jing* 精), and utilize that essence to perform bodily functions. Good nutrition is when the food can be fully transformed and used. We should become strong from it, with the Managing *Qi* (*yingqi* 營氣) flowing steadily and un-obstructively inside the meridians, and the Protective *Qi* (*weiqi* 衛氣) making a good shield on the outside of the body. When the body is cold, it is too weak to transfer essences to the right parts of the body. The essence gets stashed away in all the wrong places, and you get these lumps and humps.

She walks over to the queen mattress where I sit, and hammers a few times on my right upper arm. "Does that hurt?" she asks, "You think that's just muscles? Too much egg in your diet. I can smell scrambled eggs."

Her explanation for a hunched back is that people often accumulate excess and unwanted essence and *qi* in the hollow spaces between bones and tissues. The accumulated storage would eventually push all the bones to a slight displacement that causes soreness and pain. She hammers directly on top of these spaces, which expels the filler in that space, and thus reduces the hunch. Then she relocates the bones and joints to their proper positions. She first experimented this theory on her own grandmother, and it worked. The technique has since flattened many hunched backs in the Chinese ethnic community in San Francisco too.

Dr. Zhang does not identify herself as a psychic, but it became apparent as I got to know her better that she relies heavily on her extra senses to diagnose and heal. She gets more than olfactory hints of where and what the "food congestion" is in a patient's body. When she hammers on the body, she not only smells the food (sometimes fresh, and sometimes rotten), but sometimes sees the shape and even quantity of the food as well. The congestions are not always just food in origin. Sometimes the congestion also exists as a gush of cold air, a foul but non-food smell, or even a vision of mist or spirit jumping out and at her. She describes these sensations quite precisely as she hammers, and constantly asks the patients and other visitors if they also sense them. Perhaps she often has visitors who have extra senses like her, but unfortunately, I am not one with such a gift.

She claims to also be able to see the interior organs—when she is focused, she can see the colors and the shapes of the organs, and if there are abnormal growths. When she does pulse diagnosis, she communicates with each of the meridians, "I get a knowing of the quality of the *qi* that runs in the meridians, and what might be the problem." She gives a few examples:

> If you have too much alcohol or pharmaceutical drugs, or eat bitter-tasting vegetables like mustard greens and bitter gourds, the *qi* gets very poisonous, and there is a prickly touch to it. Sometimes people who have chemical residue in the body, that gives this numbing kind of touch, but there are other causes to numbness too. And people who consume too much grease, there is a touch for that grease in the system too. People who eat out too much and have a lot of trans-fat and reused oil in their diet, the grease feels like pellets. Those people who eat a lot of meat, oh especially lard, pork is so cold and lard is bad for you, lard feels thick and smooth, but very heavy. What is the worse situation though, is when the body is so malnourished that the meridians are too weak for me to read. Then I have to start strengthening the body for the meridians to at least be able to talk to me.

For those who are cold and weak, she recommends a diet with lots of sesame oil, ginger, and white peppers. She believes that most vegetables are too cold for the body, even after they are cooked; heavy doses of ginger are necessary to compensate. For patients who are on the strengthening diet, she prescribes herbal tonics cooked with various beans, and places a ban on fruits, which she considers to be too cold for the climate in San Francisco. She is also very specific about the type of pepper that one should consume—she insists that black pepper and other peppercorns are poisonous and should be avoided, while white pepper is gentle and warming.

A deeply devout Buddhist who cultivates with daily *qigong* meditation and chanting, Dr. Zhang says that she calls out to Bodhisattva Guanyin[9] for help when she encounters ghostly spirits that sometimes reside in the hollow spaces inside her patients' bodies. "The bodhisattva would come lead the ghosts away, so that they don't linger or stay," she describes.

Since Yiguandao followers often cultivate and claim to possess extrasensory vision, Dr. Zhang says she was told by some of her patients and friends that she emits light. She thinks that ghosts only try to get next to her when she sleeps and when the light is dimmer. Once when she woke up, a ghost was trying to leave the room in such a hurry that she rattled the glass window.

She feels that most practitioners don't cultivate enough to deal with these *han qi* (cold *qi*), evil *qi*, and ghosts. Patients often don't know how to get rid of them. When asked if she is capable of sending the ghosts away, she answers, "yes, of course" with confidence. She says it only takes calling for Guanyin, and Guanyin always comes whenever she is requested for help.

"Cultivation is extremely important," she explains in the context of encounters with ghosts and "coldness,"

> *Han* is just coldness, but sometimes that can hurt when it intrudes into the human body. Sometimes *han* from a patient can enter me and cause pain in my body. It feels like a knife stabbing, and I'd need to sit there and rest for awhile, and try to use *qigong* meditation to get rid of that coldness.

Then she explains how coldness and ghost, although experientially similar, are not the same thing:

> Ghost (*gui* 鬼) is different; it's a presence. Sometimes I actually see them and know what they look like, and sometimes I only know that it's a ghost and not just coldness. When a ghost enters the body, even after you get rid of it, there is still damage left behind that needs to be healed. Once a ghost jumped into my chest area, and I immediately felt pain. It felt almost like a heart attack . . . but really more like somebody stomping right on my chest. I asked Guanyin to lead the ghost away, but I was still in pain for three days until the wound healed.

She is fearful of such ghostly invasions into her body, but still feels obligated to help her patients who suffer from the influences of ghosts:

> It's a professional hazard, because even if I know that a ghost is inside the patient's body, I still need to help expel it. When ghosts intrude my body, because they literally squeeze into my body, it causes pain, often in my rib cage, or on one side of the body. So they jump out from the patient when I hammer down, and they leap and try to intrude into me. They look for a spot in my body that has weaker *qi*, and just jump. *Qigong* cultivation creates a shield that prevents intrusions, but when people are tired or malnourished, there are weaker spots. This is why we need to eat well, sleep well, and cultivate our protective *qi*!

I expected spirit healing to be something she started to practice in China, but she actually tells me that she rarely saw ghosts when she was in China. It was only when she moved to the United States that she started to encounter them often, both clinically and in her personal life. "My theory is that the weather in San Francisco is cold, damp, and foggy, and that is very *yin*, causing ghosts to exist." She nods as if to agree with herself. "Maybe people worship the spirits more in San Francisco . . . you know we couldn't really worship spirits in China. Here people are serious about worshiping ancestors and ghosts and gods." It is an interesting perspective considering that Dr. Zhang rarely ventures outside of the Chinese ethnic community, and socializes mostly in Chinese temples.

"It is OK to see ghosts . . . I am used to them now. I even saw my dog stay with me for a whole month after he died." Her countenance suddenly softens. "I chanted a lot of sutras to help him move on. I still chant so that maybe he could be reborn as a human next time. And that would be a very good thing."

RECAP: PSYCHIC TCM

For this group of TCM practitioners, their psychic abilities are essential for their clinical practices. They use TCM as the framework to create a space where they can best utilize their special gifts. The three practitioners position themselves in clienteles that have differing degrees of acceptance toward psychic modalities.

Tara innovatively utilizes a dowsing rod to examine her patients to arrive at TCM diagnoses. Also, as a fertility specialist, she incorporates psychic and energetic level communication, healing, and protection techniques in conjunction with standard TCM fertility treatments. Her open-minded and often desperate (to conceive) clientele embraces her unique approach. She does not hide the fact that she is psychically sensitive, and liberally uses New Age spiritual techniques to meet the needs of her patients more holistically.

In contrast, Charles hides his psychic abilities from the patients. Although he acquired the psychic abilities naturally rather than through cultivation, the resulting heightened sensitivity to people and energies became an important resource for not only his clinical practice but also his personal life. Clinically, the psychic abilities help him with diagnosis, but not in healing. Chiropractic and acupuncture are his treatment modalities, which make his practice seem "normal" to his patients.

Dr. Zhang does not have an acupuncture license, but her practice is legal because she uses only manual techniques and prescribes only herbs and diet regimens. The choice of building a patient base in the Yiguandao community allows her to accentuate the psychic aspect of her healing. The Yiguandao followers are familiar with the Daoist ideas of cultivation by meditation and diet. Furthermore, spirit possession has traditionally been an important aspect of Yiguandao rituals, where mediums perform spirit writings to transmit messages from the deities, and to provide answers to questions from the religious community. In the diversely composed general Chinese ethnic population in the Bay Area, members of the Yiguandao community have already chosen to affiliate with a tradition that values spirit cultivation as essential to the religious identity, and spirit possession as one of the main ways to communicate with deities. Individuals with heightened sensitivities or psychic abilities are highly respected in this community. Furthermore, reverence for Confucian virtues includes respect for elites. Dr. Zhang, even without formal medical credentials, is respected for being a self-educated healer who is well-versed in TCM vocabularies and theories.

Although psychic healers like Tara, Charles, and Dr. Zhang only represent a very small percentage of TCM practitioners in the Bay Area, many more TCM practitioners do recognize and tap into the spiritual dimension of their clinical practices. For some, working so closely with their patients helped them develop not only interpersonal connections but also energetic connections; through clinical experience, the healers sometimes find themselves having an embodied knowing about the conditions of their patients. Furthermore, the traditional Chinese culture, both medically and generally, conceptualizes the human body as including not only the physical, the ethereal-material (as in the life force or qi), but also the spiritual, which connects to the patterns and processes of the cosmos (more on the classical Chinese view of the body in chapter 12).

NOTES

1. Personal interview, May 15, 2008. The interview was conducted in English.

2. Wolfgang Paulus and Mingmin Zhang, "Influence of Acupuncture on the Pregnancy Rate in Patients Who Undergo Assisted Reproduction Therapy," *Fertility and Sterility* 77, no. 4 (2002): 721–24.

3. See website of American Board of Oriental Reproductive Medicine (ABORM) Certified Practitioners http://www.aborm.org/ABORM_certified_practitioners.html (accessed July 9, 2009).

4. See "The ABORM—Approved CEU Courses" http://www.aborm.org/certification/approved_courses.html (accessed July 9, 2009).

5. Personal interview, May 16, 2008. The interview was conducted in English.

6. Personal interviews and clinic observations, December 6, 2011, and December 13, 2011. Observation sessions were also conducted at the massage clinic in the Yiguandao temple on November 22, 2011, and November 29, 2011. The interview and clinic observation were conducted in Chinese, and quotes were transcribed then translated into English by the author.

7. Yiguandao, sometimes also known as Tiandao 天道 (Heavenly Dao), is a syncretic tradition founded in China in the late Qing dynasty. Currently, Yiguandao and its spin-off communities have private and public shrines in eighty countries. Recognizing Buddhist, Confucian, and Daoist lineages as different phases of the dissemination of the Heavenly Dao, Tiandao teachings attract Chinese ethnics with their emphasis in the preservation of Confucian ethics and rituals while using the familiar Buddhist and Daoist interpretations of religious activities.

8. Toisan (or Taishan 台山) is a county in the Guangdong province where many, especially the pioneer, Chinese immigrants came from. The Toisan dialect is similar but distinguishably different from the more general Cantonese dialect used in Guang-

zhou and Hong Kong. Toisan speakers among the Chinese ethnics affiliate with each other through the shared dialect and special local cuisine.

9. In Chinese Buddhism, Guanyin is the bodhisattva, or deity, of compassion.

EIGHT

Going to the Culturally Authentic

The practitioners in this chapter are not only interested in the spiritual, but they believe that the "spiritual" (defined very broadly) has always been part of traditional Chinese medicine. So they look for sources where a spiritual dimension is in the medicine: by immersing themselves in Chinese culture, by learning to read and translate the medical classics in original Chinese, and by following teachers from China.

RAFAEL (LICENSED ACUPUNCTURIST IN PRIVATE PRACTICE; PROFESSOR AT TCM SCHOOL)[1]

I met Rafael in the Chinese language class he teaches at a local TCM school. In the Bay Area, where there is no lack of practitioners who speak Chinese as their mother tongue, I was a little surprised to see a non-Chinese instructor teaching a Chinese language class that focuses on traditional Chinese medical vocabulary. Rafael is actually impressively fluent in Mandarin Chinese, and reads in both modern and classical Chinese. This is rare among Caucasian American practitioners in the Bay Area, where most know the Chinese language to the extent of key medical terms, names of some acupuncture points, and names of commonly used herbs and formulae.

The beginning of Rafael's journey to traditional Chinese medicine was inspired by the acupuncturist who treated him, whom we will call Larkin here. A Jewish American, Larkin learned traditional Chinese medicine in Taiwan, and spoke fluent Mandarin Chinese. Not only was Larkin very interested in the spiritual dimension of the medicine, he combined Orthodox Judaism with his understanding of traditional Chinese medicine. His synthesis of the two systems is so interesting that he is invited to give a talk annually at University of California, Berkeley. Rafael followed in

Larkin's footsteps, and travelled to Taiwan to learn more about not only traditional Chinese medicine, but also Chinese language and culture. Larkin remains Rafael's mentor, and shares a practice with Rafael today.

So Rafael's training in traditional Chinese medicine started in Taiwan, where through some personal contacts he found a job working in an herb shop in Taipei. He only knew a little bit of Chinese and a little bit of traditional Chinese medicine, but as he was interested in the medicine, the local customers were even more interested in him, a white guy working behind the counter of the herb shop. The customers were so intrigued by the foreign helper that they went in to see him, but ended up buying herbs. He asked many questions while working at the herb shop, but with customers constantly rolling in, the resident herbal doctor could not really provide him with systematic learning. Furthermore, he realized that the Chinese medicine he was learning was not what he expected:

> I was first exposed to Chinese medicine here in California before I went to Taiwan, and one thing that attracted me to Chinese medicine after studying it was the whole psychological and spiritual component, which I'm sure you will run into during your research when you talk to Westerners who come to Chinese medicine, because it's a fascinating part of the medicine for us. It's not in our Western medical paradigm, so the idea that the body is a holistic whole, you know, mind-body, mind and spirit, and [that] it's there present in the medical system is really fascinating. And a lot of Western practitioners, because that's what sparked their interest to start with, they like that aspect of the practice, so they spend a lot of time with their patients, talking with their patients.

However, once he got to Taiwan he had a revelation:

> In Taiwan I went to many different Chinese doctors just to see what they were doing, because I was curious. But from the Asian standpoint of practice you don't go into all that emotional stuff and spiritual stuff. The deepest advice I ever got from any of the doctors I went to go see was "*Ni xiangtaiduo le! Buyao xiangtaiduo!*"(你想太多了! 不要想太多! You think too much! Don't over-think so much!)

Without the formal training to be an apprentice, Rafael had to visit practitioners as a patient. He understood too little Chinese at the time to comprehend most of what the practitioners were saying, and the practitioners did not think a Westerner would be interested in their medical knowledge. Through a connection, he met a spirit healer who had a vibrant patient base:

> Dr. Hu was my *taichi* instructor's father. He was about eighty-four when I met him, which was in 1998. . . . He was a [spirit] medium, and he was a very devout Buddhist, his whole family and he had an altar right in the center of his clinic, which was in his home, which was a *pingfang* 平房 (single-story house). It was like an old traditional house

in Tainan 臺南,[2] and while he was seeing his patients, people from their spiritual community would come in to *baifo* 拜佛 (pay respect to Buddha) and light incense and . . . it was very interesting. Now I would try and hang out with him as much as possible but he only spoke Taiwanese. So that was a big limit, but he was very inspiring to me.

After a few years of immersion in the Chinese language, Taiwanese culture, and daily practices of traditional Chinese medicine, Rafael came back to the Bay Area for formal training. He first intended to attend a Chinese program; unfortunately, the school he wanted to attend ended its Chinese program before he even started. His fluency in Chinese still gave him the kind of learning opportunity that the English-only students did not have:

> There was one teacher at school . . . she's very much into the *Yijing* 易經 and into Chinese cosmology. I followed her for a couple of quarters when I was just back from Taiwan as an observer. We used to talk in Chinese, and she would talk with me about Chinese cosmology and these big cycles of time when Chinese cosmology—it was very interesting stuff, astrology.

Perhaps because of his unique entry point into traditional Chinese medicine, unlike most English-trained practitioners who find the spiritual dimension missing in the Communist-cleansed TCM, Rafael believes that there are always implications even in the textbooks:

> From day one in theory class we would talk about the way Chinese medicine looks at the human being as this whole, this dynamic whole which includes in their presentation mind and body. Of course in Chinese we talk about *shen* 神 and that's an important aspect of our experience as human beings, and you have to take that into account when you are treating somebody. But I don't think from the way we were taught it's necessarily a spiritual aspect of a human being. I think it's the more ephemeral aspect of *qi*. The *shen*, so *jing qi shen* 精氣神, they are all different gradients along the spectrum of *qi* in its most physical form, which is *jing*, and the most ephemeral form is *shen*. So it's there but it's not from a religious/spiritual perspective.

"What do you mean by religious or spiritual perspective then?" I ask. Rafael takes a deep breath, and goes into lengthy explanation:

> There's this idea from Sun Simiao 孫思邈[3] that intention guides the breath, breath guides the *qi* and *qi* guides the blood, so I'm sure that in that quote, what starts the process is *yi* 意, that's the intention. So that's getting very explicit at the whole body-mind connection, and you don't even have to understand that at a spiritual sense at all. You could just understand it in a psychological sense, which fits in really well with modern traditional Chinese medicine or how it's taught [in the schools here]. But even that was not really a big part of our training. It would be mentioned very quickly in class, of course the mind impacts the

body and the *shen* is this multifaceted kind of aspect of human organism that just doesn't include . . . well it includes many parts of consciousness . . . but we never went into it deeply.

In his opinion, modern TCM emphasizes too much on the physical aspect of the person:

It's only been three years that I've been practicing, and I don't have tons and tons of background under my belt. But one of the things that has stood out for me in this short time I've been practicing is this mind-body connection. Now that I've actually been practicing and working with patients it actually takes my breath away sometimes to see the connection.

He sees the connections most clearly where the pathologies are most severe:

I have a couple of patients who are quite unstable emotionally, and their physical condition mirrors that instability in their pathology perfectly. Another beautiful thing about Chinese medicine is the consciousness issue—back and forth from the internal organs. Consciousness is everywhere in the body, not just the brain, so perhaps it's the physical problems that are leading to the emotional instability, but even asking that question is a wonderful question to ask.

From the question of the connection between the physical and the emotional, Rafael finds himself exploring into the connection between spiritual philosophies and medical practices as well:

I'm just becoming more aware of how these tiny little thoughts are like seeds, and I guess this kind of gets into the Eastern philosophy and spiritual practice, although it's even present in the Western spiritual tradition. The importance of thought and how we use our mind, and even in the book of Genesis, in the beginning there was the word, logos, and from that all creation issued forth. So I'm getting a deeper appreciation for that, and I guess that would start to get into some ways where I see that spirituality can be a part of Chinese medical practice.

He attributes the search to his Catholic upbringing and his later break from the Catholic tradition:

I was raised Catholic, but then I was lucky to study in Rome for one school year. I was twenty years old and reading Marx and Neitzche, all these Western philosophers. So at a certain point I was like, I am not Catholic anymore, this is a joke.

The break [from Catholicism] grew over the course of a few years, seeing some of the democracy in the Catholic Church, seeing some of the hypocrisy. Living in Rome and being right near Vatican, and seeing the wealth of the church, and just thinking of all the injustices in the world then. You know, as a twenty-year-old I was upset, and there isn't much room for nuances to understanding some of the compromises we make as we become adults, and institutions are the same way. So one day I saw the pope leaving Vatican, and he was in his Mercedes and I thought, that's it, I quit.

Ending the religious affiliation actually started Rafael on his spiritual quest:

> I made a conscious decision to study all the world's religions. I started reading the Buddhist scriptures, the Hindu scriptures, studying Native American spirituality, for probably more than a decade I was steeped in that, and I started meditating. I had a Hindu meditation teacher, but he was very eclectic. He said, you don't have to be Hindu or Buddhist to meditate, because every spiritual tradition, Muslim, Christian, Catholic all have a meditation tradition, they call it something different.

The idea of faith traditions sharing a certain truth prompted him to not only examine what the commonality is, but also to articulate what he thinks that truth is:

> We are not our mind and we are not our body, but there's something deeper than both those things. That is eternal. The mind is constantly changing, the body is constantly changing. What is it that changes? So that just absolutely fascinated me. I guess I considered myself sort of a Buddhist Hindu for a while (chuckles).

But the experiences eventually led him back home again:

> When I was in Taiwan I was going to a lot of Buddhist temples and lighting incense and meditating and doing *taichi* in the courtyards and the temples, very nice experiences. But at a certain point I realized that everything that I appreciated about those traditions is also in my own tradition that I was raised in.

That's when Rafael revisited the Catholic tradition, but read the Christian mystics:

> It's all there! It's the same basic material—we just have to be willing to let go of some of the labels and some of our closed mindedness. I guess it was after I got interested in Chinese medicine that I've come back to my Catholic faith. I'm a practicing Catholic again but I consider myself a Catholic Buddhist.

He came around full circle, and it seems like an inclusive circle. He sees the same emphasis across traditions—constant changes as the law of nature:

> Mind and body are part of this manifest world that is constantly changing, like all the manifestations in the *Yijing* work on the level of mind and body. But there is something deeper than that, which if we learn the laws of nature like it's talked about in Daoism or *Yijing*, or even in Catholicism, there's this idea of natural law. If we come to know those laws and I see this as a big part of Chinese medical practice, in helping my patients understand how to live in tune with the seasons, how to

understand the way the *Yinyang* theory works, striving for balance in our lives, physically and emotionally. The more we come into aligning with that, the more the mind and body come into this state of this balance, the more we are able to hear that little voice inside that comes from that place.

Spirituality, Rafael argues, is therefore an important tool in medicine:

If we're intending to practice it or to receive treatments on that, deepest level is about discovering that place in us that changes.

Himself embracing an eclectic approach to his clinical practice, Rafael observes a wide range in how much his patients are open to the full scope of TCM—not just the healing modalities but also the body-mind connections and the daily practices. He is respectful of what the patients want in the therapeutic relationship:

I see some patients that come in and are totally open to all aspects of what Chinese medicine has to offer, and they're very excited about it, and want to cook herbs, and they want to hear all about the theory behind the practice, and they are fascinated by the whole thing. They are fascinated and they believe, it's like they've got this intuitive sense like, oh yeah, there is something good here.

Other patients are not as enthusiastic:

Other patients come in and I can tell they are very skeptical and it's their last resort, they've been to a lot of MDs and they haven't got any help, so they're like OK let's try Chinese medicine. So they don't want to cook their herbs, even taking herbs is inconvenient, the powder tastes bad . . . so there's a real wide range.

Currently, Rafael's personal cultivation practices include doing Wild Goose style *qigong* (*dayan gong* 大雁功) three to five days a week, and yoga on the other days. He also recently started to do some Tibetan Buddhist visualization meditation. He shares his explorations with his patients: "When I practice *qigong*, I feel like I embody the *yinyang* in my body . . . those patients of mine who want to try, I invite them to experience that too."

ALISON (LICENSED ACUPUNCTURIST IN PRIVATE GROUP PRACTICE; PROFESSOR IN TCM SCHOOL)[4]

Alison is a very busy multi-tasker: besides private clinical practice, she teaches a handful of courses in one TCM school, works in the school as an administrator,[5] participates in ongoing studies and translations of Chinese medical classics with a cohort of enthusiastic practitioners, and is the mother of a one-year-old child. In what sounds like an inevitably hectic life, Alison brings about calmness that grounds but does not sacrifice efficiency. She speaks with a comforting voice that can put anyone at ease, but the substance of her speech is always intelligently organized and clearly articulated. Despite her youthful appearance, when I attend her classes in TCM Theories and Counseling, her suaveness in delivering the materials and in inviting the students into participation comes across as a result of abundance of teaching experience. Most notably, her teaching style transports me back to my days as an undergraduate in psychology; I feel right at home, and immediately suspect that she has an unusually strong background in psychological counseling.

When I sit down to interview Alison, she confirms my speculation. For eight years, she was a volunteer counselor for a local free clinic, where she trained other counselors. She said with a grin:

> I came with a lot of experience! And in [the] free clinic there's all kinds of people coming in. And my sister is a therapist; that is always helpful. Thought about going to school in that, but that's not really how I want to interact with people, and I always wanted to do acupuncture. So I ended up doing all the prerequisites and gone to [TCM] school. I've never regretted that.

Whenever the practitioners say that they "always wanted to" do what they do now, it usually implies that they spent many years harboring the wish to do so. Like many other Caucasian American practitioners I interviewed, Alison also ventured on other paths and travelled to many places before coming to terms with the "always wanted to" option:

> When I was in college I met this woman who was an acupuncturist, and I got acupuncture from her. She was just so, I was like, I want to be like you when I grow up! She was so cool and so great, and I was studying Tibetan Buddhism and she had also studied Buddhism for a long time, and she taught me some Tibetan before I went to live in India. She used to do translation for a lot of the Tibetan teachers coming through.... She was just awesome and from that time on I just, in the back of my mind, I know that this is one thing that I'd like to do.

Nonetheless, Alison first chose to apply to graduate programs in Buddhist studies. She got accepted to several schools, and was already preparing to attend one of them. Something inside her made her hesitate:

> A month before I was going to go, I just wasn't feeling right about it. A neighbor of mine said, if you don't know what you want, ask your dreams. That night I went to bed, and I was like, OK, I'm going to ask my dreams to give me some sort of guidance here. And I had this dream that I was rushing down this hallway, I was overloaded with papers, they were like flying all over the place, there was a whirlwind around me, I was really stressed out and nervous like late for something. I thought I was going to a big lecture hall, I opened this door and there are all these people meditating in there with a teacher. It was so calm. I was like, what am I doing? I don't want to be approaching

> Buddhism this way, with this anxiety and academic work. I want to just be in it, doing it. So I decided not to go to graduate for Buddhist studies.

After years of working in counseling, Alison finally enrolled into a TCM school in 1995. She felt that her school truly prepared her for clinical practice, and she was ready as soon as she was licensed. Her life experience working with a diverse population of patients in the free clinic may have helped prepare her as well. Her teacher and mentor from TCM school invited her to join his practice. It is a group practice that includes acupuncturists and massage therapists, who not only share the clinic but also come together as a mutually supportive cohort. She had previously rented another clinic space not from this clinic, and she felt that something was "energetically wrong" with the space. Others in this current clinic cohort share her view on the energetic aspect of the treatment space. The like-mindedness of a group seems to be supportive in itself, and Alison observes the working arrangement becoming a trend:

> More and more I see people leaving school and starting community acupuncture clinics, it's a nice trend I think, it's good to work together. It definitely helps to have a few people rather than doing it all alone.

Juggling work and caring for a young child, Alison says she has not been so diligent in her Buddhist practices nowadays, but sees her experience as a practicing Buddhist as important in informing who she is:

> There is a certain thing about . . . in terms of Buddhism or whatever you want to call it, that it is just about consciousness. Whether I'm standing in line in the bank or whatever I'm doing, I'm trying to have peaceful quiet time and have consciousness, and pay attention to thoughts going by and not be attached. Bringing that consciousness to everything I do rather than having a separate time for doing that, that is what I mean that I don't "practice" as in sit down and make a space for it. It's part of my life and who I am.

That awareness of consciousness also informs her clinical practice and treatment style:

> Even every time I walk into the [treatment] room, like I'm rushing around doing these things, and I'm going into the room to take needles out, put needles in or something, I'll always like . . . ahh (long sigh) . . . take a moment before I open the door. Just ground and let go of everything, so I can really be present without all these gobbly-gob going on.

She also thinks of health in terms of being conscious. Sometimes she talks about this consciousness aspect of health with her patients:

> [We talk about] how we are thinking, how attached we are to our thoughts or our emotions, that can end up stagnating our *qi* or blocking . . . like obscuring our consciousness, obscuring our heart and soul. So then we won't be able to receive information from the universe, in

Chinese medicine they call it "the spirit of heaven guiding us." If we fill up our mind and our heart space all the time, then we can't be open to receiving. It is that reception that gives us, that really makes us perceive our world in a more real way. And we are able to perceive in a healthier direction. Whether we want to call it the spirit of heaven guiding us, or open to the universe providing us, however one wants to define it. All that comes into being conscious and open.

Besides being conscious and open, Alison also continually educates herself in her understanding of the medicine by studying and translating classical Chinese medical texts. Back when she was a student in TCM school, there were only ten to twenty hours total of classes on these medical classics, which she did not enjoy at all. However, she is now part of a small study group that meets regularly to translate and discuss medical texts written in classical Chinese:

> We are reading the *Suwen* and trying to translate it ourselves. We have an amazing teacher from France who guides us in it. I have learned more in doing that, about the basics of this medicine and what it's all about, than I have ever in all my school and my practices. I feel like, taught properly, done properly, reading the classics can be the most exciting and inspiring, amazing work ever. But it's not taught that way.

To Alison, this has been not only informative but actually fun.

> I love languages; it's something I'm totally into. One of the things I love about the Chinese language is there'll be a character, and it has all these meanings, and in this kind of very European way, because my grandparents were from Europe, it's like what I associate with them. . . . I find myself with this tendency to want to say that's bad or that's good. Translating things is like, there is never a judgment on anything, it's just . . . even when we translate "stagnation," that's not bad or good, it just IS. I've been enjoying how much . . . there isn't judgment in Chinese characters and words and . . . it's like an expression.

She feels that the current TCM school curriculum, at least at the school where she teaches, does not give enough time and consideration for the students to appreciate the Chinese medical classics:

> I think the [current assumption is], oh you already get the basic concepts. I mean, *yinyang* theory . . . I have two to three hours to teach that. Five elements theory, two to three hours to teach that. Then it's done, and we are onto everything else. A lot of that has to do with how much materials have to be covered in a short time.

As a graduate from the same time-limited curriculum that she is teaching right now, Alison cannot help but point out the irony:

> The funny thing is . . . if people get to spend a year studying just those things, everything else would just fall into place. It puts everything into the proper context. Acupuncture theories and all the details suddenly

make sense in the way that they don't as much when we skip over all that stuff. This is what I learned from this self-learning experience.

GEORGE (PROFESSOR FOR CHINESE HERBOLOGY AND CHINESE MEDICAL CLASSICS IN TCM SCHOOLS)[6]

George is the only informant in this study who does not currently practice clinically; besides teaching in the classroom, he supervises in the school herbal dispensary. Most practitioners, even if they teach or supervise in the TCM schools, find the teaching salary insufficient for the high living expenses in the Bay Area. Furthermore, doctors (as mentioned before, TCM healers are considered doctors in the Chinese cultural context) are highly respected in the Chinese ethnic community, but usually only if they practice clinically. George lives in Santa Cruz, where living expenses are lower, and currently commutes to teach in two TCM schools full-time. For the past fifteen years, he has taught in Chinese and English programs in four different TCM schools in the Bay Area.

To my surprise, George says that he had only rediscovered the true beauty of the Chinese medical classics in the past five years. Like many TCM practitioners trained in Mainland China, he was trained in scientific TCM that emphasized the traditional medicine's compatibility with biomedicine; George calls it modern TCM. Even when he was teaching courses on Chinese medical classics, he did not find himself really understanding the theoretical framework in classical Chinese medicine. When he first arrived in the United States, he taught in a TCM school in Texas, where nobody else wanted to teach the classics:

> I've taught *Shanghan Lun* (Treatise on Cold Damage Disorders) for many years. When I first started teaching *Shanghan Lun*, I was in a school in Texas. Nobody else wanted to teach the course because they thought it was too difficult. I was new, and I had to eat. By the time I arrived, everybody else had already picked the courses they wanted to teach, and I taught anything and everything, because I had to survive.

It was difficult for George to teach *Shanghan Lun* at first. However, after teaching it for a few years, it got easier:

> It was like reading the Bible for me; when I first read the Bible, it was very hard for me to understand too. Every time I taught the course on *Shanghan Lun*, I understand the book a little better. Then as I felt that I understood it better, I also realized that there were many things in there that I couldn't understand. The closer I got to the text, the more confused I was. I had many questions, but didn't know where to look for answers.

In search for answers, George spent most of his semiannual trips to China in libraries and bookstores. He especially sought books on how classical medical texts were newly interpreted:

> I wanted to know who was doing this type of research, and what they found. One day I came across this book called *Thinking about Chinese Medicine*, by an author named Liu Lihong 劉力紅.[7] Later that guy actually got invited to lecture in our school. When I read that book now, I know there are a lot of errors in it. But back then, that was exactly what I needed; it was fortuitous.
>
> Encountering that book . . . it was like a door opened up for me. After that, I was on a conscious path to explore more on classical TCM. There is so much to learn, and it's all so very interesting. What I thought I knew about in the past . . . I was merely circling outside the real door.

After entering the "real door," George wanted to explore more, and beyond just *Shanghan Lun*:

> After I came to California, my first course was also on *Shanghan Lun*. By then, only talking about *Shanghan Lun* wasn't satisfying anymore. I had to also talk about *Jinkui* 金匱 (Jinkui Yaolüe 金匱要略; Synopsis of Golden Chamber), and the Inner Classic as well. To get to the core of [classical TCM] we must talk about the Inner Classic. But the Inner Classic is very difficult to talk about, very difficult. Even now, I can't say I have completely mastered the Inner Classic, but I have a better sense of the main discourse. So when I consider the main issues, the terrain is less bumpy. Years ago, I wouldn't be able to explain the content [of these classical texts] comprehensively.

I ask how his scholarly exploration into the medical classics has affected his actual medical practice. He identifies himself as currently practicing only classical TCM and herbology. A seasoned lecturer, even though this is his dinner break, his still goes on to explain the different categories of herbal formulae in the main medical classics:

> There are two types of herbal formulae—there are the Classic Formulae (*jingfangjj* 經方) and the Practical Formulae (*shifang* 實方). All those formulae from *Shanghan Lun* and *Jinkui Yaolue* are considered Classical Formulae. *Shanghan* and *Jinkui* are actually two parts of the same book; although they are known as two of the four major medical classics, but they were both parts of *Shanghan Zabing Lun* 傷寒雜病論 (Treatise on Cold Damages and Miscellaneous Diseases). All of the formulae by Zhang Zhongjing (author of Shanghan Zabing Lun) are considered Classical Formulae, there were about 350 of those formulae. Everything else is considered Practical Formulae. All the formulae developed after Zhang, after the Eastern Han dynasty, those recorded in Tang and Song Dynasties, those are Practical Formulae. There are countless of these Practical Formulae.

Poking at the food in his microwave container, he continues without taking a bite:

> Formulae are limitless. You put these herbs together you have a formula, you put those other herbs together you have another formula. Therefore, besides the three-hundred-odd Classical Formulae, the Practical Formulae are essentially limitless. Therefore, to be a Classical Herbalist using only Classic Formulae, I use the basic principles in *Shanghan Lun*, *Jinkui*, and the *Inner Classics* to design my TCM treatments. This is for herbology only. It is impossible to practice acupuncture according to the classical texts.

"How about acupuncture then? Does anyone practice only classical acupuncture?" I asked. He continues,

> *Shanghan Lun* speaks very little about acupuncture. Furthermore, we don't have the same kind of needles. We use stainless steel needles now; they didn't have stainless steel in the ancient times. The needles we use now are extremely thin and very smooth. Ancient needles can't be made with this level of intricacy. I've seen models of ancient needles, they are much thicker, and the surface is not smooth at all. The acupuncture of that era, we can't reproduce the same effects of their treatments. Those needles must induce very strong reactions [in the body]. The needles we have now are increasingly thin and smooth, so smooth that you can't see scratches on it even under a microscope. They spray a thin layer of coating on the stainless steel needles, making it even smoother.

Besides the technological differences, he also pointed out the likely theoretical discrepancy between ancient and modern acupuncture:

> The acupuncture points are also different. Although there are historical records of acupuncture practiced in the ancient times, and although the Inner Classic dedicates much of its content to acupuncture, the truth is that the locations of the standardized acupuncture point locations and the processes related to acupuncture, those don't come from the four major classics. Classical descriptions of acupuncture we see today come from later compilations and interpretations, from the acupuncturists in Sui and Tang Dynasties. The general directions of the meridians are the same as the Inner Classic, but the actual acupuncture points are different. Therefore, we can't apply classical theories on modern acupuncture. The points are not the same, and the tools are not the same.

As I have mentioned in chapter 3, the medical classics have only been increasingly incorporated into the TCM curricula in the past few years. The revival coincides with George's personal discovery of modern interpretations of classical theories, and he had chosen to become an expert of the new trend. This combined with his opinion that TCM practitioners should have extensive knowledge in the four Confucian classics (see chapter 3), makes it clear that he recognizes the power and authority in being culturally and textually authentic in TCM.

He finally takes a bite of his food. He chews very slowly, swallows carefully, and says,

> Classical TCM is the real deal. It took me a long time to realize that, but I've taught these books many times now. I'm getting better at explaining the classics, and the students are getting better at learning them too.

RECAP: POWER IN THE CULTURALLY AUTHENTIC

Mostly as a response to the lack of systematic and evidence-based knowledge production within the TCM profession in the Bay Area (see chapter 3), practitioners in this group seek "culturally authentic" sources to enhance their understandings of the medicine. Rather than depending on the local TCM schools and continuing education programs (which are incidentally also accessible to all competing practitioners in the area), these practitioners circumvent the "middlemen" and try to tap into sources of knowledge more directly.

The authenticity in Rafael's case is in his extensive exposure in the Chinese cultural and linguistic context. The traditional mode of knowledge transmission—through following the master and learning more through watching the master practice—gave him not only medical information, but also a model for clinical treatment and self-cultivation. He enters a mode of concentration and focus in the clinic, which helps him connect to his patients on the energetic level.

Alison and George both approach the question of authenticity by exploring the classical medical texts. Allison, being non-Chinese, has to slowly learn how to translate the classical texts in order to have better understandings of the nuances of a condensed form of Chinese that was written hundreds, if not thousands, of years ago. The translation process is tedious and slow, and the texts are difficult to understand without the culturally embedded references that most Chinese elites are equipped with. This is probably the reason why George suggests that the Confucian classics should also be taught in TCM programs, because he is fully aware of the cross-textual references that have historically been crucial in how Chinese elites educate themselves.

George's decision to completely abandon modern TCM in lieu of classical theories is an interesting one. His interpretations and incorporations of classical theories provide a non-biomedical perspective in understanding and framing TCM practices. By focusing on the classics, TCM could hold up as its own system, rather than having to constantly reference biomedicine as the standard. On the other hand, George also recognizes that the acupuncture aspect of the classics may not be as useful today, considering the advancement in the tools and the inconsistency in the point locations. However, I wonder if the same critique can hold true for herbology as well—do the herbal formulae have the same potency with the modern technologies used in processing them? And might humans today, with our much more polluted environment and with chemicals in our daily lives, react to the Classic Formulae differently?

I ask the above questions not only because opponents of TCM often attack the medical system for the lack of controlled studies to prove its actual efficacy. My observations of many TCM clinics in the Bay Area and survey of TCM practitioners across California suggest an interesting pattern—that there seems to be a trend of TCM practitioners envisioning a controlled environment that promotes healing holistically. In the next chapter, we will see how TCM practitioners in the Bay Area conceptualize and construct the environmental aspect of their clinics, clinical practices, and their patients' daily lives.

NOTES

1. Personal interview, November 7, 2008. The interview was conducted mostly in English, but Rafael occasionally used some Chinese terms and phrases to clarify his ideas. When he did use Chinese terms, they were noted and translated into English by the author.

2. A municipality in southern Taiwan.

3. Sun Simiao 孫思邈 (581–682) was an herbalist, doctor, and Daoist priest in the Sui/Tang dynasty. He left behind a wealth of herbal formula in *Beiji qianjin yaofang* 備急千金要方 (Essential Formulae for Emergencies Worth a Thousand Pieces of Gold) and supplemental volume *Beiji qianjin yifang* 備急千金翼方 (Supplemental Formulae for Emergencies Worth a Thousand Pieces of Gold). As a Daoist practitioner, he also authored texts on cultivation techniques and healing rituals.

4. Personal interview, November 12, 2008. The interview was conducted in English.

5. By the time this chapter was drafted in July 2009, Alison is no longer holding any administrative position in the school.

6. Personal interview, October 18, 2008.

7. See Lihong Liu, *Thoughts on Chinese Medicine* (*Sikao Zhongyi* 思考中醫) (Taipei: Jimu Wenhua Publishing, 2004).

NINE

Healing, Environment, and Lifestyle Changes

In traditional Chinese cosmology, the world consists of Heaven above, the Earth below, and humans in the middle. The universe and all beings share the basic life force, *qi*, and all are governed by the same set of principles that not only transcend, but also correspond across, categories and dimensions. Aspects of the natural world and different dimensions of human existence are categorized according to the shared principles of *yinyang* and five elements, and are juxtaposed. Across dimensions and existences, those that fall under the same categories share a common set of characteristics, and resonate. In short, human beings are connected to nature because they correspond with the patterns of Heaven and Earth, and resonate with the cycles and movements in the environment.

Developed with such cosmology as its backdrop, TCM theoretically identify the human body and nature as not only interconnected but also synchronized.[1] In the richly diverse Californian context, ecological discussions on nature preservation and sustainable living are often informed by multicultural sensitivities and pluralistic spiritual understandings. In this chapter, I will show how TCM practitioners find themselves inevitably contributing to the popular discourse as healers who mediate between Chinese and American cultural systems. In turn, the ecological discourse in the TCM clinics emerges from this cross-cultural attempt to demonstrate the understanding of human existence as an integral, synchronized part of the great cosmos. In order to heal the person, the healer must heal more than just the physical body; but by healing one body, we might also be healing the environment simultaneously.

TCM, as a medical system that theorizes based on the assumption of the transcendent nature of *qi*, provides the space for dialogues in the clinical setting by recognizing an inherent connection between human and nature. With the TCM practitioners, from the physical sensation of *qi* movements and the experiences of enhanced healing effects after their self-cultivation, there is often a deeply felt connection with and appreciation for the environment.[2] From the perspective of many of these TCM practitioners, the environment must be protected not only because humans are part of it, but because humans inevitably resonate with every aspect of it by sharing the same essential substance, or breath—the *qi*. As healers participating in the Californian ecological discourse, the practitioners not only focus on restoring and maintaining the health of their patients, but also engage themselves in actively improving and preserving the environment, which contributes to the general well-being of all existences within it. The efforts manifest in several dimensions of TCM practitioners' clinical practices: from the attention to details in creating a transformative clinical environment, to cultivating themselves to provide more effective healing, to interpreting environmental concerns through the lens of TCM theories, to educating the patients into assuming responsibility in maintaining healthy lifestyles.

HEALING BY THE ENVIRONMENT: TRANSFORMATIVE CLINICAL EXPERIENCES

From clinic visits, I found that there is a wide range of individual styles among the TCM clinics—some are sterile and functional, some are quiet and minimalist, some are warm and filled with the scent of herbs, some aim to relax with dim light and soft music, still others reflect the particular aesthetic preferences of the practitioners in charge. Despite the varying presentations, there is a shared attention to the clinic ambience. At the TCM school's community clinics where new practitioners were trained, the group treatment sessions also provided patients with hot mint tea (which filled the room with a comforting fragrance), indirect and dimmed lighting, soft background music, and whispering practitioners.

The peaceful, tranquil, and sometimes spa-like clinic environment is more popular among the non-Chinese practitioners. With the Chinese ethnic practitioners, many try to emulate the sterile, hygienic image of biomedical clinics, while some others try to invoke a sense of energetic vibrancy by having lots of live plants in the waiting room, or by displaying *fengshui* or ethnic-themed decors. Many (but not all) of the TCM clinics I visited have a small water fountain, a fish tank, or sometimes both. Within the Chinese cultural context, having a fountain or fish tank in the clinic makes perfect sense. Objects that contain flowing, moving water are popular ritual objects to have in businesses—water signifies wealth, and having flowing water in a business is believed to have the energetic effect of making customers, who bring with them money, flow in. With the popularity of *fengshui* in the United States, there is no doubt that even some non-Chinese practitioners would use the flowing water objects as auspicious decorations, if not as ritualistic tools that are believed to cause energetic transformations financially.

Another question I asked in the survey was this: what first impression do the practitioners want the patients to have upon arriving at their clinics? This is an open-ended question, and respondents listed their own adjectives; 50 percent of the respondents listed "professional" as the impression they want their patients to have upon entering their clinic. But that was only the second highest ranking. Adjectives that suggest the atmosphere of a "sanctuary"[3] (safe, healing, calming, relaxing, soothing, and so on) ranked the highest at 58 percent. Related to "sanctuary" are adjectives that suggest "peacefulness" (peaceful, still, and quiet) which were also listed by 30 percent of the respondents (see Appendix, Table 15). Among those who listed "sanctuary"-related adjectives, 85 percent of them were Caucasian American practitioners. This trend was also seen in those who listed "peacefulness"-related adjectives, where 81 percent were Caucasian American or non-Asian. When I correlated those who wished to have a water fountain and/or fish tank in their clinic with those who list either or both of "sanctuary" and "peacefulness"-related adjectives, statistics showed that twenty-nine out of the thirty-five respondents (83 percent) in the overlap between groups were Caucasian American practitioners.

These simple statistics suggest that the Caucasian American practitioners may have a different symbolic understanding of the water fountain and the fish tank from their Chinese-American colleagues. In the Chinese context, the goal of having business-enhancing ritual objects is to produce a state of *wang* 旺, a kind of prosperity with flamingly high energy and fast pace that conjures an image of a noisy, crowded marketplace. Although Chinese practitioners may not necessarily want their clinics to be noisy and crowded, no one would object to having the effects of the *wang* energy reflect on the account books. Whereas the Chinese would see the flowing water as symbolic of moving and vibrant energy, the American interpretation of the flowing water is of serenity and calmness. The quiet, relaxing, almost spa-like atmosphere is nothing like what the *wang* energy would produce; "sanctuary"-like is energetically gentle and tamed whereas *wang* is energetically aggressive and upward. The *wang* state suggests that to the Chinese, a clinic is primarily a type of business, but to the Caucasian practitioners there is a spiritually nurturing undertone to the ideal clinic atmosphere.

Alison, a Caucasian American practitioner and a TCM theories instructor at the local TCM school (see chapter 8), shares her perspective on the importance of the clinic atmosphere:

> It's not something I can put into words, but I can say, it's the flow and movement in the space. The other people in the space. There is some-

> thing about what energy is left there by people or brought there by people. The colors. The amount of light. Plants. All of those things. They are all small things in a way, but as a whole . . . I've had people who, I can remember recently someone came in the wrong time for their appointment. . . . She said, just sitting in your waiting room, I sat and I felt so peaceful in there that I just felt better when I left. Even though, you know, she just sat in there. That is really important to me.[4]

In short, the healing process can start from the moment a patient steps into the clinic. It may be without a direct treatment session with the practitioner; on the other hand, the clinic ambience as the creation of a practitioner resonates with the intention of the practitioner.

If ambience is indirect presence or extension of the presence of the practitioner, practitioners also cultivate themselves to amplify their healing efficacy in the clinic. By cultivation, I include practices that are commonly known as "cultivation practices," where the shared goal of the activities is to cultivate the person, whether it is physically, emotionally, psychologically, or spiritually. When I approached practitioners with the concepts, they listed exercises they do to make connections between the physical and the spiritual, between outer and the inner, between the individual and nature, and so on. Some listed sports regimens, and explained that the physical exercises help them get "more in tune with their own bodies." Secular sports can possibly serve the same purpose as many of the more physically oriented cultivation practices.[5] Although many expressed that they do not necessarily tell patients about their personal cultivation practices, when asked how relevant these practices are to their clinical practices, only 10 percent who responded think they are not relevant. 72 percent of the respondents think that these practices are either very helpful or extremely important to their clinical practices.[6]

Estelle, a young Caucasian American practitioner who is building her patient base by working in two clinics, shares how her personal cultivation helps with her clinical treatments:

> I realized if I do have a daily spiritual practice I would feel a lot better—more centered and calm. So I can't honestly say that I follow one religion; I definitely don't go to church or anything like that. I'm not a big believer of that. But I do have my daily meditative spiritual practice, and I do yoga a lot. To me that's like my spiritual practice, because before and after [treatment sessions] I meditate for like ten minutes. To me that's when I feel the most. . . . I guess when what people feel like when they're doing their religious practice, which is light and solitary.
>
> I need to feel centered to be able to be there for my patients fully. I know the days I'm off: maybe it doesn't come across to the patients, because my nature is . . . people think I am very together and grounded. But if you're having a bad day, it is so hard to be present.[7]

Rafael, the Chinese-speaking Caucasian American practitioner who teaches medical Chinese in the local TCM school (see chapter 8), establishes the connection from the perspective of oneness. He shares a memorable lesson from his mentor:

> [My mentor] said to me, "So one thing that you need to start to think about and cultivate is this very very clear realization that when a patient comes into the clinic, and they're sitting there in front of you, that it's just one of YOU in the room."

The oneness of the practitioner and the patient facilitates the healing practices. In his clinical practice, he tries to keep that conception in mind:

> Just yesterday, when I was seeing patients, I thought about it at a few different points with two different patients. I remembered that the awareness came in, and it felt like the whole treatment just went smoothly from that perspective. It's a beautiful way to approach life, especially in the medical context.

He further explains why the approach is significant to him, even when he recognizes that he does not fully comprehend the process:

> I guess it is sort of like meditation in a way you just visualize it, or you have that intention. I don't know how much of it comes from my previous exposure doing spiritual practices, but it's just a question of constant practice and cultivating our mind and refining our vision, and the way we experience ourselves in the world. It's just kind of a split second of remembering, and it's totally mysterious, and I don't understand it. It's just this cool concept, but I feel like there is something to it, like when I do remember that, I feel like the whole treatment just unfolds in this much more natural, don't know if it is spontaneous. Yeah, it just feels like it goes better.[8]

Several other practitioners also say that self-cultivation helps them perform more effective treatments and stay energized for the long workdays. By connecting to nature and tapping into the universal *qi*, practitioners become grounded, centered, and energetically resourceful for the needs of their patients. By connecting to the patients, the practitioners become channels through which the patients benefit from not only the treatment but also the healing effect of the environment.

QI POLLUTION AND THE ENVIRONMENT

Mostly through practice and action, many TCM practitioners connect themselves to nature, their environment, and their patients to reinforce their healing. Beyond training their patients to become more aware of what they *take in* from nature—for example, ingesting only healthy food and dietary supplements suitable to one's specific constitution, and avoiding herbs polluted by pesticides and harmful minerals—some practitioners also discuss with their patients what goes back into nature. Besides topics on recycling, energy conservation, and lower car emissions, the most unique type of "pollution" talked about in the TCM clinics is *qi* pollution. The logic goes as follow: since we all share the universal *qi* and are connected by it, then the diseased or negative *qi* (*bingqi* 病氣) can also be contagious even if the illness itself is not pathologically infectious. Therefore, if that particular *qi* is not properly neutralized, it can become unwanted pollution to make more people and the environment sick.

Practitioners who cultivate regularly strengthen themselves to protect against such *qi* pollution. In fact, some Chinese ethnic practitioners have explained to me that the reason why physical cultivation is especially important for a healer is that one must strengthen his or her own protective *qi* (*weiqi* 衛氣) to stay healthy while spending so much time in the clinic with patients. A few Caucasian practitioners who have backgrounds in visualization meditations say that they visualize a transparent barrier between them and the patients.

Sally, who is the director of the medical *qigong* program in a TCM school, uses *qigong* healing regularly in her private clinical practice. I asked her if she does anything to protect herself from diseased *qi*, or if she has strategies to cleanse or neutralize a space that has been occupied by a patient who may have very potent *qi*. Sally describes her procedure for keeping the treatment rooms and her clinic free of potentially injurious *qi*:

> When I treat a patient, I also create a vortex in the room that sucks the bad *qi* out of the room. It's like a tornado that directs diseased *qi* away and keeps the room clean and ready for the next patient.[9]

Sally is not explicit about how such a vortex is created, but the concept sounds a lot like a kitchen vent that expels smoke and odor out of the house. The implication of such a procedure becoming part of her clinical routine is that it is likely that it is also part of the standardized treatment procedure in medical *qigong* practices in the Bay Area, or at least for students who attend the certificate program that she directs.

Ashley, another practitioner who incorporates *qigong* healing into her acupuncture practice, uses large pieces of jade and blessed blankets from her *qigong* master to neutralize diseased *qi*. When I observed at her clinic, she showed me pieces of jade with black spots—signs of diseased *qi* being absorbed by the jade. She said it takes a while for jade to neutralize itself, whereupon the black spots disappear. I mentioned to her a common practice to neutralize stones and crystals energetically: by placing them under running water. Ashley disapproves of the practice: "The water will take away the diseased *qi*, but then it goes down the drain and goes into the rivers and the ocean. We shouldn't be polluting nature that way."[10] Instead, Ashley prefers to rotate the jade pieces for them to neutralize naturally, and to chant upon the blessed blankets to help them clear from the diseased *qi* they absorb during treatments.

The environmental awareness is sometimes a mixture of Californian sensitivity and the Chinese classical understanding of the juxtaposition

Healing, Environment, and Lifestyle Changes 153

between nature as the macrocosmic version of the human body, and the human body as the microcosmic version of nature. George provides here a classical Chinese interpretation of a modern environmental concern, the greenhouse effect:

> The source of greenhouse effect is petroleum, because it creates heat. What does petroleum corresponds with in the human body? In the human body, the essence of kidney (shenjing 腎精) is like petroleum. The essence of kidney is the most precious in the human body, because it cannot be regenerated. It comes from one's parents, and however much your parents gave you is what you get. It will not regenerate, and only gets consumed [overtime]. That is why people die; when the essence of kidney is completely consumed, then one dies.

Using Chinese classical correspondence logic (see more in chapter 11), he explains why the kidney and petroleum can be understood as parallels with shared characteristics:

> Kidney corresponds with water. The color that corresponds with kidney is black. The function of kidney and water are to store. All the characteristics of petroleum are identical to the characteristics of the essence of kidney. They are both black, they both flow, and they both store, and they cannot be regenerated. And the essence of kidney is also an energy source. And this type of energy theoretically should be stored underground. The scientists don't know why it is hidden underground. But this stuff cannot come out [from the ground]. I didn't know what ill effects there'd be for [petroleum] to leave the ground, but now we know it causes the greenhouse effect.

He points out that it is natural and therefore "healthier" for petroleum to stay underground:

> [Petroleum] should be hidden and stored underground. It is relatively healthier for [petroleum] to stay underground. Of course it will eventually age, just like the human body. Some people are healthy and free of diseases, but they eventually die too. The planet Earth is the same way. But [to keep petroleum where it should be] can possibly prolong its life.

Similarly, it is natural and healthy for the human body to properly store the essence that fuels the whole body system. The relationship between the classical Chinese understanding of essence (*jing* 精) and the modern conception "energy" is very much like how petroleum can fuel a flame:

> For the normal human body, energy is fire. This fire is not like *shanghuo* 上火 (inner heat rising), but means that we all have energy. When we sleep, this fire is hidden, and it hides in the *yin*. When we wake up, the *yangqi* comes out again. Whether a human can stay alive depends on whether this fire is there.

In other words, just as a small pilot light is always kept alit in a gas stove, the human body has a "fire" that stays hidden to make sure that the proper conversion process is always ready to keep the body functional. A healthy body, however, should be fueled by the essence derived from regular intake of nutrition, rather than the emergency reserve of kidney essence. Otherwise, the human body will eventually get ill for operating against the general, universal way.

Following the same set of natural patterns, George explains how burning petroleum fuel rather than wood for fire is just like burning the emergency reserve of kidney essence:

> Where does this fire come from? In principle, fire comes from wood, because wood generates fire. Summer must come after spring, and so making fire from wood is a great situation because wood regenerates and grows back. But here [with petroleum] what do we use to make fire? We are using water [because petroleum corresponds with water]. [In the cycle of five elements], there is wood between water and fire, and now we skip the wood to make fire directly from water. The benefit [of using petroleum] is that the energy that is produced is high, because the fuel efficiency is high. But the side effects are starting to show. In terms of the human body, that is like shortening one's life span. In terms of the world, the planet Earth grows warmer. More problems will appear, because the planet is already ill.

George does not offer a concrete solution for how environmental problems can be solved, but he believes that since the same principles are shared between the human body and nature, scientists should look for inspirations in TCM theories.

Some practitioners also promote a healthy lifestyle and environmental awareness by providing reading materials in only those genres in their clinics. For example, one practitioner only has yoga, vegetarian diet, and healthy lifestyle magazines in the waiting area; on her receptionist counter are information on nutritional supplements and occasional flyers for lost pets in the local community. Another practitioner stated bluntly: "I don't want trashy magazines polluting my patients while they wait for me to fix them."[11]

CULTIVATION AND LIFESTYLE CHANGES

When I inquired the TCM practitioners about their perspective on the causes of disease (and symptoms, for those who separate disease etiology from symptoms), two trends emerged from the collected data: 1) most practitioners believe that there are multiple causes of disease in the human body; and 2) instead of the classical TCM etiology, the most popularly identified causes of disease are actually a mixture of biomedical and holistic categories. Unhealthy "lifestyle" is the most emphasized cause of disease (88 percent), followed by the "disharmony between body and mind" (79 percent). These two chart toppers are main concerns in holistic medicine, where proper lifestyle and the harmonious integration of dimensions such as mind, body, and spirit are believed to lead to overall health of a person. The next two most popular causes are biomedical categories: "pathogens" (65 percent) and "pollutant and chemicals" (60 percent). Even "blockage," a key word in the energy paradigm, only gets identified by 48 percent of the respondents. The classical TCM etiological categories such as "excess/deficiency" (33 percent) and "wind" (32 percent) are not as highly recognized as the prior terms.[12]

In other words, TCM practitioners in California focus on how their patients carry themselves and relate to the environment ("unhealthy lifestyle and disharmony between body and mind") more than using the classical TCM disease explanations of internal imbalance ("excess/deficiency") and external invasions ("wind") or the biomedical diagnosis of infections ("pathogens") and poisoning ("pollutants and chemicals"). Although it is recognized that some patients are ill due to reasons that they have no control over, a commonly held position among practitioners is that the patients can achieve better health if they assume responsibility to achieve it through cultivating better habits and connections between the physical and beyond-physical, between the self and nature.

When patients seem open to the idea of self-cultivation, sometimes practitioners recommend that their patients pick up a practice too. Among those practitioners I talked to, many share their cultivation methods with their patients, mostly informally. A few teach more formally: one practitioner teaches yoga classes in the studio behind her clinic, another teaches free *qigong* classes in the local park on the weekends, yet another opens his home kitchen to patients and teaches them raw food preparations (see the case of Dr. Hsieh below). Here we see the transfer of responsibility of healing from the practitioner to the patients. The responsibility, whether it is in the form of practicing to cultivate and strengthen one's *qi* and connection with the universal *qi* or to prepare health-enhancing food, is to make positive changes in one's lifestyle.

DR. HSIEH (LICENSED ACUPUNCTURIST; TUINA SPECIALIST; RAW FOOD ADVOCATE)[13]

Dr. Hsieh is a Taiwanese immigrant practitioner who uses mostly *zheng-gu* and *tuina* techniques in his practice. In the South Bay, where Dr. Hsieh lives and practices, the competition for practitioners specializing in *zheng-gu* and *tuina* can be quite fierce. Not only is he competing with other licensed acupuncturists, there are numerous massage therapists with and without certifications who also compete in the niche of "health maintenance." A third force that just joined the niche market is the blossoming foot massage shops. These shops that specialize in "foot washing" (*xijiao* 洗腳) have become popular in China in the past few years. Chinese transnationals are always keen to see business opportunities in the Chinese immigrant community, and this is an example of providing a type of service that is trendy in China. For very affordable fees compared to whole-body massage ($15 to $20 compared to $50 to $120 per session), Chinese foot massage includes a foot soak in herb-infused hot water and massaging of the feet, often up to the knees.

Dr. Hsieh is a talkative healer. During his treatments, while patients undergo painful (fortunately very quick) adjustments, he bombards them with Buddhist teachings at the same time. During his treatments, Dr. Hsieh must bare his feet and stand firmly on the ground. He explains that his cultivation has led him to be able to sense and see not only the movements of bodily *qi*, but also energetic entities that lurk around. Although self-identifying as Buddhist, his stories reveal a Taiwanese folk Daoist worldview where deities sometimes come forth, through their presence or channeling through him, to aid in his healing. He entertains patients with miraculous stories of treatments involving exorcisms of sorts, where by his *qigong* he drives away harmful ghostly entities. Those who sit on the side waiting for their turns gasp at his vivid descriptions; whoever happens to be under his merciless therapeutic hands grunts and whimpers accordingly.

Dr. Hsieh's business thrives because he does more than just *zhenggu*. A vegetarian and a Buddhist, Dr. Hsieh challenges his patients to a complete lifestyle change: raw vegetarian diet, regular *qigong* exercises and hiking trips, and Buddhist cultivation if possible. As a seasoned chef, he provides free cooking demonstrations for his patients, in his home kitchen, on how to make salads and smoothies. He claims that he can cure cancer with just a raw vegetarian diet alone, and his acupuncturist friends have tried to explain to him that such claims can have negative legal ramifications. Even with patients who are not severely ill, he claims that a vegetarian diet would make his work easier—not only would that help the patient get rid of excess and toxic waste from the body, but also tendons and muscles would become softer for easier manipulation.

Currently, Dr. Hsieh's clinic is located in a strip mall. The store space that he uses as a clinic was previously a dance studio. Rather than remodeling the space, he kept the dance floor and open layout and only uses makeshift stations for treatments. Several times a week, he has a group of regular patients help him clear the floor, and they have exercise sessions, and occasionally even karaoke and ballroom dance after. He also organizes hiking trips on weekends to encourage his patients to get in touch with nature.

"You need to change your ways to be well, and nature has a lot to offer," says the doctor as he offers me yet another glassful of his thick, mossy concoction, "I promise if you follow my diet plan and go exercise with me a few times a month, you will feel much better!"

MASTER LIN (FOLK HEALER AND TEA MASTER IN PRIVATE PRACTICE)[14]

In a very industrial section of San Francisco, Master Lin's center is located above a bike shop. I knock on a small door that is colorfully decorated with Buddhist symbols. The door opens to a steep, creaky staircase. Up, up, and a turn, I am greeted with the deep vibration of a Tibetan horn in the background music. Behind a tea table sits a man, probably in his forties, with eyes that are both warm and penetrating. He is quite good looking, with an air of mystery, or dare I say, exoticism, about him. Donning a delicately embroidered yet visibly worn jacket that looks like the work of the minority tribes in Southwest China, Master Lin shakes my hand and continues with the conversation he is already engaged in with three other visitors sitting around the tea table. The master speaks near-perfect English, with only a slight hint of a Chinese accent, which adds to the general intrigue.

I sit down on a low wooden bench, and Master Lin pours me a small cup of *Pu-erh* tea. I look past him and see an intricately woven bamboo screen behind him, and a Daoist dust sweeper (*chenfu* 塵拂; usually used as a ritual object) hanging on the screen. The dust sweeper, with a handle made with silver and mother-of-pearl, is the most beautifully made one I have ever seen. A classical Chinese style side cabinet also exudes old-world charm. Master Lin pours a second cup of tea, which is a different *Pu-erh*, for all five of us visitors to try. Sitting next to me is a musician with a full head of impressive dreadlocks. Next to the musician is a young, clean-cut, yuppie-looking coffee shop owner. Another young man works in the organic produce store nearby. On the other side of me, a younger man sits in a relaxed lotus position. He says that he is an engineer, but his furrowed, thick brow somehow makes me think of Rumi's poems.

Master Lin doesn't refer to himself as a doctor or healer, but as a tea master. He trades tea from all over China, and trains students as professional tea masters who "train others and spread the arts of tea." Over the many cups of tea, he tells stories of his childhood in a rural village in Southwest China, where they had very few medicines besides tea, and they would boil tea leaves, add a lot of sugar to it, and drink that as medicine for small ailments. He tells of a life where the village people sit around all day drinking tea and chatting, just like what we are doing. We are all enchanted by his stories, his soft-spoken yet clear voice, and the enigmatic persona.

Behind the bamboo screen, the room opens up much wider into a treatment room with four treatment tables, side by side, with no dividers. Patients flow in as we chat, and continually fill all the treatment tables. Master Lin leaves us only very briefly to check on the patients, but his student mostly takes care of the treatments.

After much casual chatting over tea, Master Lin takes us on a tour around the center. Behind the open treatment room, there is a tiny little ladder, the kind that takes you to the attic in an old house. Master Lin takes the lead and opens a plastic trapdoor upward. On the top of the roof is a camping ground: six tents make a circle, with a laundry washer, a sink, and an old bathtub in the middle, with nothing over them but the sky above. We are invited to peek into the tents. Every tent has a sleeping bag or a mattress, and some personal items. An especially large tent has a queen-size air mattress in it, and three shelves jam-packed with books. "That's my personal library," Master Lin points out with pride. The tents are not completely enclosed, and I catch myself shudder just trying to imagine how cold it would be sleeping in there in those windy, freezing cold San Francisco nights.

"My students stay here, and I sometimes do too," Master Lin smirks, as if he is sharing with us the greatest secret of the universe. "You see the freeways there? They look like rivers. People think we are in a lousy neighborhood. I say we have great *fengshui*!"

His students pay $600 a month to stay in one of the rooftop tents. When there are vacancies, students from the nearby TCM school have also lived in the tents; apparently, a place to stay for $600 a month is hard to come by in the city. The residents have the option to pay another $250 a month for food. Master Lin would take them on grocery shopping trips, and teach them how to cook and eat healthily. He insists that the students who want to train under him must live a "complete lifestyle." Those who cannot afford to pay him for the board, training, or treatment in cash can work for him in exchange. He himself has an exchange type arrangement with the landlord, who is also the owner of the bike shop: in exchange for using the second floor and the roof, he gives the landlord's family and employees free treatments. When he makes profits from the operation of the center, he also helps pay for the mortgage of the place. In essence, it is a commune.

Curious about what Master Lin does for his treatments, I ask what I should expect if I were to schedule an appointment for myself. He describes that he takes cash only, and the initial treatment, which includes detailed pulse reading, the design of a personalized one-hundred-day treatment plan, and two weeks' worth of herbs, would be $300. Licensed acupuncturists in the Bay Area typically charge $45 to $150 for initial treatments, and only some of the very prestigious and senior practitioners charge more than $200, herbs excluded. Some practitioners charge more for the initial consultation, while others have a single rate for all treatments. Community clinics, which Master Lin's treatment area resembles, typically charge significantly less than clinics that provide individual treatments with private rooms. He must have noticed the shock in my eyes. Perhaps attempting to ease the blow for me, he suggests that, like some of his patients who do not have the means to pay him in cash, I can possibly make arrangements with him to do small jobs around his center in place of the treatment fee.

There are also preparation requirements before the initial treatment: for the entire week prior, the client must drink at least one liter of water in the morning and another liter of water in the afternoon. For the three days prior, there should be no animal products, wheat, or rice in the client's diet. The reason for the preparation, Master Lin continues, is to help him make a more accurate diagnosis.

With the enthusiasm and clarity of an infomercial host, Master Lin explains his treatment model:

> Do you know that the human body is made up with 70 percent water? The problem with most people in today's society is that they are dehydrated. The first thing we must do is to make sure that the body is again consisting of 70 percent water.

The daily two liters of water for the week before the initial treatment is only to prepare for even higher water intake; once treatment starts, clients are asked to drink four liters each day of herb-infused water. I am also asked to purchase alkaline test strips from medical supply stores to test the acidity of my saliva for the week before the initial treatment. Master Lin requests that his clients keep a daily record of the pH level of their saliva as a way to see progress, and as a way to emphasize that his healing is "scientific." He also asks to read medical charts and test results if the clients have known illnesses.

After the initial treatment, Master Lin's one-hundred-day personalized plan consists of biweekly visits with him where he keeps track of the client's condition with pulse diagnosis, and treats with cupping, manual manipulations, and customized powdered herbs (to be infused in the daily four liters of water). When I ask him what he means by manual manipulation, he demonstrates by quickly taking my right wrist, applies pressure on several points, and flips my hand over skillfully while maintaining continuous and penetrating eye contact the entire time.

Clients are also given "lifestyle homework" to do between clinic visits. He further suggests that after the one-hundred-day plan, clients should continue to "check-in" with monthly visits. After careful consideration, I decide to not go back to Master Lin for actual treatments. The researcher part of me wants to go back and find out more about how he practices clinically and how he maintains a booming business (it was one of the busiest clinics I have visited in the Bay Area) without a license. On the other hand, besides potentially parting with a serious amount of cash, I am not entirely comfortable with the idea of downing gallons of mysterious herbal concoctions each day for more than three months, especially when I don't have a serious enough health condition to justify potential risks in doing so.

As I was leaving, Master Lin was in the middle of pouring more tea for a tea trader friend, and discussing a plan of building a lifestyle resort near his hometown in Yunnan. "People will be away from their busy life, have healthy food, and make tea with good water. I think that is what most people need," he winks, "and I think people will like it."

RECAP: HEALING BY CULTIVATING CONNECTIONS

The "environment" in this chapter's discussion comes in two levels: one is the environment of the TCM clinics where the treatments take place, and the other is the larger environment of nature in general. TCM practitioners try to provide a transformative environment in their clinics by the hardware—layout, music, lighting, decors, and equipment, and by the software—the cultivated, sensitive, *qi*-abundant selves of the practitioners. Practitioners also engage in environmental concerns and issues outside the treatment rooms. Some use TCM theories as the vantage point to understand and interpret environmental problems. Others share with their patients methods and tips on self-cultivation to tap into *qi* in the environment, which include lifestyle changes to include more physical exercises, diet regimens, and so on.

Dr. Hsieh and Master Lin are both examples of TCM practitioners who introduce a wider range of "changes" in their interactions with the patients. These lifestyle changes reflect the holistic nature of the TCM medical paradigm—that the health of a person is not limited to only the physical body, and that to heal the physical body, there are more ways than to only use medical modalities in the clinic to treat only the physical body. In the next chapters, we will explore more on the various dimensions of human existence that TCM practitioners try to address, and how both modern practitioners and classical Chinese medical texts conceptualize human, the cosmos, and health.

NOTES

1. My usage of the term TCM includes a wide variety of practices under the broader umbrella of Chinese medicine, rather than as the equivalent of state-regulated TCM in the People's Republic of China (PRC-TCM).

2. Without using the terminology, many practitioners in the Bay Area promote what scholars of ecological discourses call "deep ecology," which is "deeply felt spiritual connections to the Earth's living systems and ethical obligations to protect them." See Bron Taylor and Michael Zimmerman, "Deep Ecology" in *Encyclopedia of Religion and Nature* (London: Continuum, 2005), 456–59.

3. This is a category I created after the responses were collected and sorted, as with all the broader categories listed in Appendix, Table 15.

4. Personal interview, November 12, 2008.

5. In my survey, only 15 out of 138 respondents either did not do any of these practices or chose not to answer. The rest of the respondents checked from one to

many of the items on the list as activities they regularly practice. More than half (53 percent) of the respondents say they try to "get in touch with nature" regularly; it is interesting to note that this is popular even with people who do not have other "practices." Sitting meditation is the next popular activity (37 percent), with *qigong* exercises (31 percent) and *taichi* exercises (28 percent) to follow. "Praying to God, Allah, or the Goddess" is regularly practiced by 25 percent of the respondents, while "communicating with spiritual beings and forces" is also favored by 25 percent of the respondents. There is a clear trend of regularly practicing to become more in tune with the environment, the cosmos, and within oneself; in other words, we can safely say that the TCM practitioners are doing a fair amount of spiritual cultivation in their private time. See Appendix, Table 15.

6. Percentages come from my 2006 survey.
7. Personal interview, September 3, 2008.
8. Personal interview, November 7, 2008.
9. Personal interview, January 29, 2009.
10. Personal interview, October 2, 2009.
11. Personal interview, April 19, 2008.

12. The numeric data is collected through my 2006 survey. A similar trend was observed in my formal interviews.

13. Informal interviews and interactions between June 2008 and May 2010 were conducted entirely in Mandarin Chinese.

14. Informal conversations and interactions, September 12, 2008. The conversations were conducted entirely in English.

TEN

The Happenings in an Acupuncture Clinic

In the previous chapters, I have outlined the historical and cultural context of TCM in the Bay Area, and introduced the modes, experiences, and personal narratives of a range of TCM practitioners. This chapter is a more comprehensive view of the clinic of one practitioner. Ashley is a Caucasian American practitioner who has close relationships with her Chinese ethnic mentors. I observed in Ashley's clinic for three months, and was allowed to observe during treatments with the permissions of the patients. Although there are many personal styles in how TCM clinics operate, Ashley's clinic is representative in the general spirit of TCM in the Bay Area—eclectic and utilitarian in practice, and soothingly comfortable in its atmosphere, yet at the same time keenly responsive to market competition.

THE LOCATION

The commercial plaza has a surprisingly beautiful and spacious central courtyard, with some flowering plants and even outdoor furniture for those who work in the plaza and the customers to enjoy the sun and fresh outdoor air. Facing the courtyard is Ashley's clinic. The corner unit has large full-length windows that allow light and the view of the courtyard into the clinic's waiting area. A jingling bell on the door announces the arrival of patients into the clinic. In the small waiting area sit two rocking chairs. A Tibetan Buddhist *tangka* graces one wall, while other decorative items are charmingly situated by the windows. The two front treatment rooms are also artfully decorated, with items such as an elegant kimono and framed print from a classical Chinese text on the wall, and antique

Chinese porcelain trays on top of bamboo woven side tables. Soothing music fills the space but is never distracting. The receptionist, Kathy, answers the phone politely and professionally with her signature British accent. Beside the reception counter, Ashley's dog Rumba crouches with his eyes half open. Patients love Rumba; everyone greets and pets him, sometimes even before greeting the humans in the clinic. Some patients request that Rumba be in the treatment room with them; others ask to take Rumba out for a walk before or after their appointments.

THE PRACTITIONER AND THE PRACTICE

Ashley's personality is much like her clinic: pleasant without cliche, engaging but not overpowering. A petite woman with shoulder-length grey hair, Ashley has no makeup on but glows naturally. A *qigong* practitioner for longer than she has been practicing traditional Chinese medicine, she not only utilizes *qigong* clinically but also teaches it for free, once a week in a park near her home, and also in the plaza where her clinic is located. Her patients are encouraged to attend these *qigong* classes, but if they are not able to, she also finds time to teach them the basic exercises and movements that can benefit their particular bodily conditions.

In 1984, Ashley started to practice *taichi quan* and *qigong*. She remembers the exact moment that first opened her mind to the possibility of understanding the human body beyond the visible. One day after about six months of practicing a *taichi* movement called Cloud Hand (*yunshou* 雲手), Ashley felt a shot of lightning through her hands. Shocked and amazed like a child playing with the electrical outlet and getting buzzed for the first time, she asked her teacher what that was about. Her teacher responded matter-of-factly, "That's your *qi*, that's your energy. You can feel it and you can see it. Oh yeah."

At this transformative time, there was also another transformative person in her life. Living in San Francisco at the time, Ashley became close to an elderly man in Chinatown. The ninety-year-old Chinese man took Ashley under his wings like a grandparent, and taught her many small wisdoms in the Chinese way of life—how she should cook with certain herbs in the fall to prevent catching a cold in the winter, or eat certain food to avoid getting arthritis when she grows old. He also took Ashley to see his acupuncturist, who not only treated her with needles but also prescribed more herbs for her. After downing the bitter herbal brews for a week, Ashley felt healthier and "like a new person."

As if bodily experiences and personal influences were not quite enough, there were also constant visual hints coming her way. When she drove her mentor back to Chinatown, she always passed by an acupuncture school. She got inspired:

I thought, hmm . . . maybe in my last life I was an acupuncturist. And then I thought, why not this life? Why don't I take one or two classes and I can treat myself anyway? And that was it. It was like I opened up this treasure chest, and there are jewels to be found every day.

She took action, enrolled into a TCM school, and successfully attained her state license. As a new practitioner, she practiced with two other friends in the city of San Francisco, treating many HIV and AIDS patients in the free clinics and in their own clinic, charging them only $10 per treatment. Soon, the goodwill practice was proven to be financially unsustainable, and Ashley opened another clinic in a town on the border of the Peninsula and the South Bay. For a while she commuted between the two clinics, but finally decided to focus on her solo practice, which is also closer to her own home.

It was not easy to start a sustainable and profitable solo practice. For the first few years when she was slowly building her patient base, she could not afford to hire a receptionist, and had to run the clinic completely by herself. After more than ten years of network cultivation, Ashley can now afford to hire her part-time receptionist Kathy, who assists the general operation of the clinic—answering phone calls, scheduling appointments, ordering herbs and supplies, tidying up treatment rooms, and closing up the clinic at the end of the day. An immigrant from England and the mother of two teenagers, Kathy's gentle and loving presence also contributes to the positive and welcoming clinical atmosphere at Ashley's clinic.

Recently, Ashley also introduced two associates to her practice, a junior licensed practitioner who specializes in facial rejuvenation and fertility, and a massage therapist. Kathy schedules appointments for the associates, but Ashley does not pay the associates fixed salaries. Instead, the associates pay Ashley overhead for using the treatment spaces and equipment. The junior acupuncturist, Estelle, who is also a partner in an integrative clinic in the East Bay, says this particular working arrangement allows her to cultivate a patient base in the area without having to invest in the lease of a clinic, equipment, and human resources. For Ashley, the arrangement does not add much to her financial liability, but ensure that her patients' needs and demands are better addressed, and that the associates can care for her patients on her off days if necessary.

While many licensed acupuncturists advertise their practices, Ashley promotes her practice with a multi-pronged approach. Deeply aware of the importance of professional networking, Ashley works closely with local oncologists, fertility experts, and other biomedical physicians, and participates in several research projects in a prestigious medical school nearby. Providing public educational lectures alongside biomedical physicians not only puts Ashley's name out in the local community as "endorsed by the respected doctors," but also gives her opportunities to promote traditional Chinese medicine to the local community. In 2012, she also officially started to take clinical interns from Stanford University Medical School. The medical students shadow her around the clinic, but without a license to practice biomedicine or acupuncture, the interns are not allowed to practice acupuncture, as it is considered an invasive procedure.

Understanding the power of face-to-face interactions, Ashley throws parties at her clinic, where she invites her patients and those who own businesses or work in the same plaza to come in and have some food, chat, and enter a drawing for one free treatment.

With healthy nibblers and herbal beverages on the buffet table for everyone, Ashley converses with her guests as a good party hostess. Rather than leading a session of line dance or Macarena, she demonstrates some beneficial *qigong* movements. Her massage therapist associate, Sandy, gives free five-minute chair massages on the side. Business cards are on the buffet table, but nobody focuses on sales pitches. On the other hand, the image of a friendly local clinic that is there when you ever need help is probably much more effective than any mail, newspaper, or internet advertisement.

Ashley's training in acupuncture and herbal medicine, which are the standard modalities covered by the acupuncture license, come from not only her TCM school training, but also continuing education courses and several senior Chinese practitioners who are long-time friends and mentors. Most notably, for the past decade or so, Ashley has studied under a *qigong* master from China who claims to be the lineage holder to the Emei 峨嵋 school. Mount Emei, located in the Sichuan province, is one of the four sacred Buddhist mountains in China (its patron bodhisattva is Samantabhadra or Puxian 普賢 in Chinese)[1] and is historically known for its martial arts training. More practical than religious, Ashley's master has a curriculum that consists of *qigong* practices, healing techniques that utilize *qi* infusion, Buddhist mantras, sounds, and blessed ritual objects such as an embroidered blanket and items made of jade. Most significantly, the master teaches a medical system that is theoretically consistent with the common traditional Chinese medicine, but with innovative techniques and technologies that often seem to come from Daoist and folk religious sources. It is essentially a wider scope of medical practice that includes ritual and energetic healing in the repertoire. The master does not self-identify as Buddhist or lecture on Buddhist ideals. Instead, he labels his *qigong* and other practices as "cultural and scientific."[2]

As Ashley advances in course levels in her master's system, she gathers a rich array of healing techniques that she uses in her clinics whenever she deems the situation is appropriate and the patients receptive. She also continues to use other modalities and techniques that she has on hand, for example, Korean needling techniques, electronic stimulation machines, and Master Tung's points (an alternate set of acupuncture points). Sometimes, after she does regular intake with a patient and goes through strategies she has tried, she cocks her head to one side in thought, rushes out of the room to get yet another gadget, and tries it on the patient. With an undergraduate degree in fine arts, she has remained an artist at heart—the clinic is her studio and medicine is her medium.

Ashley typically sees four to seven patients in a working day, scheduling them in half-hour intervals starting from late morning or early afternoon, and ends before 7:00 p.m. Patients who come to Ashley are mostly women (a few men), Caucasian American, and middle- to upper-middle-class professionals and retirees. The area that Ashley's clinic is located in is generally well-to-do. "Sometimes I Google my patients' names and they turn out to be really rich or are pretty big in their fields," muses Ashley, "so that's really interesting." She treats her patients, even those who have become personal friends over the years, all with the same level of professionalism during the healing session. On the other hand, it is worth noting that since Ashley runs a cash-only business (she provides statements for patients wanting to make health insurance claims, but her clinic does not process insurance claims), it does take a certain level of financial ability to afford the once-a-week maintenance sessions that many of her patients come for. Perhaps $85 a session ($125 for the initial session, herbs not included) is still less expensive than spa treatments, but it does add up when it becomes an ongoing routine.

The patients at Ashley's clinic consist of a financially capable crowd, but not all are soiree-attending socialites. Among them are also young professionals who try to take better care of their bodies after stressful days of work, career women with families and children, and retirees who are busy with community activities and volunteering. Ashley's magazine basket in the waiting room only has magazines on topics such as healthy living, alternative healing, environmental consciousness, and yoga. On the receptionist counter, there are often flyers the patients bring for community events and sometimes notices for missing pets. If we zero in on the demographic, one patient's casual comment might give some hint: "I have this friend who I love dearly. . . . I love her even though she is Republican and voted for George W. Bush." And everyone in the room nods in silent understanding that such friendship truly transcends unthinkable obstacles and divides.

Of course not all of Ashley's patients are progressive liberals who are socially responsible and environmentally friendly, but individuals with this particular set of characteristics seem to make up her core patient base that stay with her practice long term. These patients are comfortable with the healing that she provides, and are mostly very open to the more radical techniques in Ashley's repertoire. Some of her patients also visit other practitioners of alternative healing regularly. Patients come in for general conditioning and preventative care, chronic pain management, stress management, and fertility issues. Most do not have "illnesses" that they would visit a biomedical doctor for, although a few with chronic conditions do have physicians they work with. Perhaps that's the main reason they come to see Ashley—so that they can prevent actually becoming sick enough to require biomedical care.

Patients at Ashley's clinic are scheduled at least thirty minutes apart from each other, and each patient spends about an hour in her clinic per visit. There are three treatment rooms, but she usually uses two of them at any given time. When a patient comes in, Ashley greets the patient and invites him or her into a treatment room. She closes the door and conducts a brief intake session where she chitchats with the patient briefly and asks how the week has been. Regular patients voluntarily check in with her on their general activities and observations of their own physical and emotional conditions. If the patient is concurrently undergoing other medical treatments, he or she would usually update Ashley at this point, but only voluntarily. After the patient has a chance to become relaxed and calmer in breath, Ashley takes his or her pulse, sometimes with the patient sitting in a chair with both feet on the floor, or lying on the treatment bed.

If the treatment requires the patient to remove his or her clothes (mostly to access acupuncture points on the back), Ashley leaves the room briefly to allow the patient time to get ready. She then places needles into appropriate acupuncture points, and leaves the room for the needles to work for twenty to thirty minutes. Meanwhile, the next scheduled patient would be due in the waiting room, and Ashley would start the second patient in another treatment room. After putting needles into the second patient, Ashley then returns to the first patient to remove the needles and finish the treatment.

Comfort of the patient is carefully attended to in Ashley's clinic. Soothing music always plays in the background, in volume that is calming and not disturbing. A portable heater, various heating pads, and blankets are readily available to keep the patients warm. On some chilly days, Ashley keeps small towels on top of the portable heater so that she can cover the patients' feet with toasty towels. Cushions and pillows of various sizes, heights, shapes, and textures are also available for the patients' choosing. The overhead lighting can be dimmed so that patients do not have to stare directly into bright light.

THE THERAPEUTIC REPERTOIRE

Depending on the condition, severity, needs, and preferences of each patient, Ashley has a sequence for utilizing her "tools in the box":

1. The very basic treatment consists of acupuncture on the standard points (points along the standard meridians), and herbal supplements are often recommended but never required.

2. If the standard acupuncture points are not sufficient, then alternative points such as Master Tung's points or Korean acupuncture tools for finding potent points are used.
3. If normal needle stimulation is not sufficient, *qi*-infused stimulation of the needles is used. Sometimes Ashley also massages along the meridian of the points she needles to enhance the flow of *qi*.
4. For cases that are more severe, negative *qi* is removed from tips of needles (still inserted in the acupuncture points) with a grab and throw movement of the hand toward a special blanket or a piece of jade, both blessed by Ashley's *qigong* master. She chants a mantra "Ami dili gonzhen hong" repeatedly while doing this movement. The blanket is sometimes used to cover an area on the patient's body that may need extra help, and blessed jade is placed under the location of pain.
5. If the spot removal of *qi* is not enough, Ashley performs a larger scale removal where she has her hands a few inches over the problem spot (usually larger area) above the patient's body, and does a sweeping movement toward the patient's leg and out into a piece of blessed jade in her hand while chanting.
6. With a few stubborn cases, Ashley also uses another technique where she produces a very loud, explosive sound with her mouth. That is to help break up the *qi* blockage.
7. For some patients who cannot tolerate direct acupuncture (severe pain or very sensitive to pain), Ashley can also do indirect acupuncture on a plastic human figurine that has the meridians and acupuncture points labeled on it. The patient is asked to see where the needles are inserted on the figurine. Patients report the sensation of a surge of energy at the actual physical location corresponding to the needled location on the figurine.
8. If after using all the physical techniques, there is still no satisfactory progress in the patient's condition, judging from the particular patient's level of tolerance toward the "unconventional" and nonphysical treatments, Ashley may recommend using astrological readings and an intuitive calculation technique to look for causes to the condition in the form of past emotional trauma.
9. Although Ashley is able to treat most patients who come to her, if she does not feel that she can treat the condition or if the patient is simply not a good fit with her, she refers them to other practitioners.

For patients who do not feel comfortable with treatment methods beyond the regular acupuncture, or are not interested in the herbal supplement, Ashley does not insist on using her extra tools. With new patients, she starts with the minimal and watches their reactions—both the progress of physical healing and their acceptance of her more radical tools. Most of her long-time patients are fascinated by and comfortable with her usage of the more spiritual healing strategies.

RECAP: CREATIVE HYBRIDITY

In Ashley's clinical practice, we see traces of several of the previously mentioned orientations. Ashley creates a healing environment that is more comfortable and relaxing than most of the biomedical clinics, but she also actively seeks opportunities to work with biomedical doctors. She incorporates *qigong* and an array of energetic techniques, astrological calculations, even psychic healing into her practice, offering "spiritual" healing for physical ailments of those patients who are open to trying new treatments. Finally, although Ashley does not devote herself to learning to read Chinese medical classics in their original form, she follows a Chinese master who teaches an entire system of esoteric healing that claims its root in the Daoist tradition.

In this complex hybridity, Ashley freely crosses the boundaries between systems of healing in search of the best, customized approach to each patient who comes to her. The patients can choose the types of treatments that they feel are acceptable and are comfortable with. On the other hand, the patients are on the expedition with her, trusting her judgment and skills to practice her own version of TCM, which is enriched by knowledge from other alternative medicines in the United States, other Asian medical systems that also use acupuncture, standard TCM and less standard TCM techniques, and techniques from Daoist and Chinese folk medicine as taught by her *qigong* master.

Ashley also creatively taps into a rich array of resources and authorities. She establishes working relationships with biomedical physicians, who not only give her biomedical endorsements, but also actively refer patients to her. She connects with the local business owners to tap into the possible human connections in the community. She invites patients and local community members to clinic parties to make personal relationships. She greatly increases her collection of treatment modalities by following a Chinese master who is a wealth of esoteric healing techniques, and from continuing education programs offered by local TCM institutions. All these efforts are investments that lead to her healing efficacy and business success.

NOTES

1. Mount Emei became a Buddhist mountain after the eighth century. Prior to that, it was known as a Daoist mountain.
2. See the Emei Qigong website: http://www.emeiqigong.us/ (accessed September 15, 2009).

ELEVEN

The Embodied Spirituality of *Qi*

Whereas English speakers greet each other with "You look great!" Chinese speakers often greet each other with something similar: "Your *jingshen* looks great" or "The color of your *qi* looks great." Good *jingshen*, roughly translatable to "good spirit" is understood as a certain vibrancy of energy that manifests outwardly. *Qise*, literally the color of *qi*, is seen as the manifestation of one's state of health by the tone of a person's continence. Most Chinese speakers, whether they are science fanatics, religious adherents, or otherwise, will likely not think of these notions as "spiritual," or as many would prefer to say, "mysterious" (*xuan* 玄), but rather, something quite physical and easily observable.

There are indeed known proponents in the TCM profession who resist anything that could possibly be unscientific or not proven by Western biomedical clinical trials. However, from conversations with practitioners in the Bay Area, I have noticed that even those Chinese ethnic practitioners who refuse to talk about the "nonsense" of superstitious/religious/spiritual are willing to talk about *qi*. Understood as the life force that permeates and is shared by all beings in the universe, in traditional Chinese medicine, *qi* is understood as fundamental to the functioning of the human body. It is the breath of life and more; all aspects of human health can only be achieved with proper circulation and balance of a person's *qi*.

WHAT IS SPIRITUAL?

There are two fundamental difficulties in talking about what is "spiritual" in the contemporary Chinese cultural context. First, the Modernization Movement that was initiated at the end of the Qing dynasty and the introduction of Communism propelled the Chinese elites into a century-long resistance against "superstitions." Many of the spiritual and religious ideas, behaviors, and practices were vehemently rejected as primitive and counterproductive to the advancement of the Chinese civilization. Those who consider themselves educated and intellectual do not take interest in the discourse on "spiritual." Although late Qing and early republic intellectuals such as Kang Youwei 康有為 (1858–1927) and his students advocated for the establishment of Confucianism as China's national religion, they were mostly interested in the social and political application of Confucian theories, and not the ritual and spiritual aspects of the tradition.

Furthermore, while the term "religious" has been conveniently equated with things that have to do with religions, or *zongjiao*, there is no consensus among scholars or my Chinese ethnic informants on a Chinese equivalent for "spiritual." Most Chinese terms used to translate the English term "spiritual" are problematic and misleading when taken out of context. Compound words that include *ling* 靈 as a component, which has the connotation of spirit, vibrant life force, magical power, enlightenment, and efficacy[1] are often used to translate "spiritual." These compound words include *shuling* 屬靈, *lingxing* 靈性, and *xinling* 心靈, among others.

Shuling, which literally means belonging to or associating with *ling*, is usually used by Chinese Christians in talking about their relationship with the Holy Spirit, which is translated into *shengling* 聖靈. Within the Chinese Christian context, "spiritual life" is conventionally called *shuling shenghuo* 屬靈生活, or life that belongs to or is associated with *ling*, or the Holy Spirit. The term is rarely used by non-Christians. *Lingxing* means literally the nature of *ling*, commonly used to describe inanimate objects, plants, animals, and other non-human entities that seem to carry with them a magical sort of enlightened intelligence, or are perceived as having profoundly vibrant life force. In the Chinese folk religious context, sometimes a giant rock or an especially old tree is worshipped for its *lingxing*, which can be due to its exceptional size or age, or whatever sense of profoundness that it conjures out of the worshippers. Animals that exhibit extraordinary intelligence or behaviors that resemble human emotions and sentiments are often said to have *lingxing*. *Xinling*, or the heart-mind spirit, is recognized and used increasingly frequently by New Agers and self-help groups in Chinese societies (yes, they do exist and are growing with incredible force) as a dimension of human life that is beyond physical but still part of the individual. Although it may first appear to be a suitable translation for the more general and inclusive understanding of "spiritual," it may or may not be adequate in covering the more diffused sense of "spiritual," which may have more to do with sensations that are physical but invisible.

Sophia, the TCM practitioner who is also a philosopher (see chapter 2), suggests the term *jingshen* 精神 as a translation for "spiritual." As part of the widely known trio of *jing qi shen* 精氣神, which can roughly be translated as essence (refined materials), life force, and spirit, essence is the core of the physical aspect of human existence, while the *shen* is the extra-physical. In its modern usage, *jingshen* as a compound word is used in terms of the extra-physical, metaphysical, and psychological dimensions of a person. In modern vernacular, it can also be used as an adjective to describe a person who is especially energetic, vibrant, and focused. Perhaps the implication is that a person with a high level of energy and focus demonstrates the state where his *shen* is actually refined.

However, in contemporary biomedical parlance, the term *jingshen* is used as the standard translation for the medical specialty of psychiatry (*jingshen ke* 精神科). Whether the Western association between psychology and Eastern spirituality is the cause or result of this particular contemporary usage of the term is probably a chicken-and-egg debate. However, I would argue that unless carefully limited within the classical Daoist and Confucian understanding of the term, the fact that *jingshen* has become an equivalent of Western psychology/psychiatry in its contemporary usage renders the term much too confusing to use generally.

Meilun (introduced in chapter 3) articulates *jingshen* and *linghun* as two different dimensions, where both are connected with what the English term "spiritual" approximates, and includes philosophy as another dimension in the mix. These are separate yet connected and possibly overlapping categories, which is Meilun's way of talking about the knowing of what is beyond the physical:

> When Chinese medicine approaches and knows (*renshi* 認識) things from the psychological/spiritual (*jingshen*) dimension, from the philosophical (*zhexue* 哲學) dimension, and from the soul/spiritual (*linghun* 靈魂) dimension, it can be very abstract.

The challenge of concretely and precisely identifying a single Chinese equivalent for "spiritual" points to the question of cross-cultural creations and understandings of categories. Through my countless discussions with Chinese ethnic informants in finding a satisfactory equivalent of "spiritual" in Chinese, it occurred to me that perhaps the question should not be how the Chinese ethnic practitioners think about the spiritual dimension of their practice. How can they possibly talk about a conceptual category if they do not have the category? Furthermore, my position as a researcher from the discipline of Religious Studies necessarily brings forward the term *zongjiao* or "religion" which many of the Chinese ethnic informants, especially those who grew up and were educated in the People's Republic of China, equate with "superstition," which is in turn the opposite of science, modernity, and everything that is powerful and advanced in today's world. They may not want to talk about known categories that they understand to be uncalled for, but does that necessarily mean that they do not think about and believe in things that may otherwise belong to the category that they have yet to know, which exists in a different cultural context?

So the million dollar question becomes: How can we talk about a dimension of human activities and conceptions that is possibly shared across cultures but are not necessarily categorized and articulated in corresponding terms?

To give a better sense of the challenge of even starting a conversation on "spiritual" in the Chinese context, let us hear how Sophia attempts to process the concept:

> Spirituality . . . as long as it's not pretentiousness, then that's fine. If that's the true spirit of this practitioner, then that's fine. You can use your spirit to engage people, with patients. A more loving, caring . . . a caring art. That is part of the practice. But that does not easily translate to knowledge. Knowledge is such that . . . for TCM, if you come in with a problem, and if this problem requires certain knowledge from TCM, I don't want to tell you that I love you and you'll be healed. This is a different level of treating the body. I love you as a patient so I will care for your problem, but I am still required to use my knowledge, how to use my judgment, how I'm going to engage you, and how to treat this problem. So that part is knowledge.

It is interesting that although she highlights knowledge as the most important aspect of approaching a medical problem, she also suggests that the practitioner must first engage with the patient with her spirit. She said the word "spirit" in English, but based on her earlier suggestion that *jingshen* should be the closest translation to spirit, she was probably using the term "spirit" with connotations of *jingshen* in mind. How does one engage with others with the extra-physical aspect of themselves? In the next section, I will use some classical Chinese sources to explain.

CLASSICAL UNDERSTANDINGS OF *QI*

In attempts to better describe what *qi* really is, Western scholars have variably translated the term into "life energy," "vital force," "vapor," "material force,"[2] and "psychophysical stuff."[3] The concept is also often considered similar and parallel to *prana* in Vedic medicine, *mana* in Pacific Islander worldview, and common English terms such as breath, energy, and so on.

As my Chinese ethnic informants emphasize and explain repeatedly, the human (and in turn the human body, if there is a difference between the two) is part of a cosmos within which everything shares the essential material of *qi* and functions according to the principles of *yinyang* and the five elements. Furthermore, regardless of ethnicities, most of my informants recognize that *qi* is an entity that spans across the physical human body and other dimensions of human experience. Even the most avid promoters of scientific TCM recognize that emotions can be treated by managing the corresponding meridians, which are channels of *qi* in the human body. This understanding is historically shared by the Confucians and the Daoists.

Confucius (BCE 551–479) was said to never talk about *guai li luan shen* 怪力亂神,[4] which has been variably translated as "prodigies, feats of strength, disorders or spirits,"[5] "prodigies, force, disorder and gods,"[6] and "extraordinary things, feats of strength, disorder, and spiritual beings,"[7] leading to the interpretation that Confucius was against topics related to superstitions. Thanks to the lack of punctuation in classical Chinese, the phrase can also be interpreted to be talking about *guaili* 怪力, abnormal power, and *luanshen* 亂神, chaotic spirit, where it is completely reasonable that nothing goes beyond what is human. To rephrase: Confucius never talks about the abnormal power of a person that is against the flow of nature that follows the principles of *yinyang* and five elements, and chaotic spirit as in the lack of calmness in the *shen* of a person, *shen* here being the visibly observable manifestation of a person's state of mind. In short, Confucius, the expert in rituals that aimed to align the human with the principles of Heaven and Earth, quite possibly was merely suggesting that we stay with the natural flow of things.

Confucius himself never directly talked about *qi*, but we know that the concept has been widely accepted and discussed by Chinese elites as early as the Spring and Autumn era (BCE 770–476). Guan Zhong 管仲 (BCE 723–645), a renowned politician and scholar, explains the most basic understanding of *qi*:

> With *qi*, there is life; Without *qi*, there is death. Living depends on *qi*. Acquire it and you live, lose it and you die. What could that thing be? Only *qi*.[8]

The Daoist philosopher Zhuang Zhou 莊周 (BCE 369–286) states similarly:

> When a person is alive, *qi* accumulates and amasses. When *qi* amasses, there is life; when it disperses, there is death.[9]

This life-giving entity is shared by all beings in the universe, as posited by Laozi Daodejing (circa sixth century BCE), another Daoist philosophical classic: "Yin and yang mold and cultivate myriad beings, but they are all born from one *qi*."[10]

Zhuang Zhou describes how *qi* gives life: "When *qi* transforms, it becomes physical forms. When physical forms move, there is life."[11]

The oldest existing Chinese medical text, *The Yellow Emperor's Inner Classics* (*Huangdi Neijing* 黃帝內經; dated approximately somewhere between BCE 450 and BCE 200), explores extensively the qualities and functions of *qi*, especially in the context of understanding human illnesses and how to heal them. It tells of how the quality of *qi* inside a person can affect his or her well-being:

> All diseases are affected by the *qi*. When one is furious, the *qi* goes upward (in the opposite direction). When one is joyful, the *qi* calms down. When one is sad, the qi dissipates. When one is afraid, the *qi* goes downward. When one encounters cold, the *qi* contracts. When one is hot, the qi discharges. When one is shocked, the *qi* is disorderly. When one is fatigued, the *qi* is consumed. When one is anxious, the *qi* stagnates.[12]

Notice both emotional and physical conditions are noted as affected by *qi*, which shows that *qi* is not limited to just making physical effects. Not only does *qi* transcend the differentiation between individual humans, but it also transcends dimensions of human existence and experiences. In fact, when one is truly synchronized with the universal *qi*, Lie Yukou 列禦寇 (exact dates unknown), a Daoist philosopher and contemporary of Zhuang Zhou, tells us that the differentiation between different senses actually disappear. One loses the physical form and becomes the heart-mind (*xin* 心),[13] which is metaphysical:

> Thereafter the eyes are like the ears, the ears are like the nose, and the nose is like the mouth; they are not differentiated. The heart-mind is consolidated, but the form dissipates, and the bones and flesh completely dissolve away.[14]

THE BODY THAT IS SEVERAL BODIES AND ONE BODY

Japanese scholar Ishida Shigeru 石田秀實 proposes that the ancient Chinese viewed the human body in a binary fashion—that there is an understanding of the body in terms of fluid, moving *qi*, and another understanding of the body as the physical field within which the *qi* would flow. He calls the former "the flowing body," and the latter "the situated body." It is a perspective of the body that simultaneously recognizes the human body as both the physical form that serves as the location or container, and the always moving and flowing *qi* that infuses the physical body with life.[15]

While Ishida's binary model provides us with a general sense of the ancient Chinese view on the human body, Chinese philosopher Hu Fuchen 胡孚琛 identifies a three-pronged model specific to philosophical and cultivational Daoist texts. There is a physical form (*xing* 形), and there is also the *qi*. On top of that, there is *shen* 神 (spirit). Hu argues that the Daoist model considered all three components essential to the human body. First, the physical form and the spirit cannot exist without each other. And most importantly, nothing can exist without *qi*.[16] This view is exemplified in the Daoist cultivational classic *Baopozi* 抱朴子 by inner alchemist Ge Hong 葛洪:

If the physical body (shen 身) is exhausted, the spirit (shen 神) will disperse. When *qi* is depleted, life is over.[17]

Jing 精, the essence of all the nutrients that nourish the body, is the fuel for the physical form. *Jing*, *qi*, and *shen* are three manifestations of the same material force, covering the spectrum from the most crude and physical form (*jing*), to the ethereal yet still physically sensible form (*qi*), to the most refined and thus immaterial form (*shen*). And because these three components are so essential, Hu affirms that all Daoist cultivation methods orient toward the three goals of training the *xing* or physical form (*lianxing* 煉形), promoting the flow of *qi* or life force (*xingqi* 行氣), and preserving the *shen* or spirit (*cunshen* 存神).[18] Daoist inner alchemists, who used their own body as the caldron, and *qi* as material to extract elixir, describe the cultivation process: First one would start with *jing*, which is the material essence of the nutrients from food. From *jing*, *qi* can be extracted. Then, from the *qi*, *shen* can be distilled. Finally, *shen* needs to be further refined until it returns to the Great Void which is the primordial form of the cosmos, before differentiation of *yin* and *yang*.[19] That would be the state of human and cosmos becoming one.

With the potential of becoming one, qualities of human are contrasted and defined by juxtaposing them with the cosmos. The *shen* component of human existence is analogized to and correlated with Heaven (*tian* 天), and the *xing* or *jing* component with Earth (*di* 地), where both Heaven and Earth came into existence from differentiation from the same primordial *qi*. Both analogies and correlations take place—not only are the humans symbolically compared to the cosmos, the human body is understood as also exhibiting identical patterns and functions as the cosmos. We can understand the cosmos and the human body by approaching one to understand the other; the cosmos is the human body in the macro scale, and the human body is the cosmos in the micro scale. This mode of juxtaposition by correspondence between macro and micro, between big and small, and sometimes even between different aspects of one being (for example, different aspects of human experiences such as the physical vs. the emotional), is a core characteristic of classical Chinese cosmology shared by Daoist and Confucian elites alike.

The first major compilation of Daoist essays, *Huainanzi* (BCE 139), provides examples of this very mode of juxtaposition:

> *Jing* and *shen* were bestowed by Heaven, and the *xing* (form) and *ti* (physical body) were responses to Earth.... Therefore the roundness of the human head looks like how sky is round; the squareness of the feet also look like earth. In Nature, are four seasons, five elements, nine directions, and three hundred and sixty-six days [in a year]; Human also has four limbs, five inner organs, nine orifices, and three hundred sixty-six joints. In nature there is rain, wind, cold, and hot; in human there is also joy and anger.[20]

Here we see a slightly different juxtaposition between the human and cosmos, where *xing* and *ti*, which are solidly physical, associate with Earth, while *jing* and *shen*, which are not solidly physical, are associated with Heaven. Classical Chinese medicine also juxtaposes the internal organs and the four seasons through sharing the general patterns of the five elements This juxtaposition then allows logical predictions of conditions and events based on the rules of five elements. However, it is more than just an assumption that this juxtaposition takes place; classical sources also offer explanations for how it works.

Confucian scholar of the Eastern Han dynasty, Wang Chong 王充 (25–97), who vehemently attacked the folk belief in harmful ghostly apparitions, suggests that *shen* 神 (spirit) is only a form of disembodied *qi*, just like water is unfrozen water:

> The way that *qi* become human is akin to how water become ice. Water freezes to become ice; *qi* solidify to become human. When ice melts it becomes water, and when a person dies, he returns to being *shen*. The label of *shen* is akin to the fact that ice is the name for another state of water.[21]

Underlying this analogy is the understanding that water and *qi*, both being materials in nature, share the same guiding principles for the processes of "becoming" different forms. Again, the notion of *shen* and *qi* as different forms of the same material suggests that the *jing-qi-shen* trio are actually consistent in essence but differ in manifestations. And indeed, the three are found to be used interchangeably in various classical texts.

Neo-Confucians in the eleventh to twelfth centuries explored extensively how *qi* can have consistent patterns across different realms, entities, and dimensions of existence. Zhang Zai 張載 (1020–1077) was the first to articulate the model that myriad beings take on physical forms because *qi* amalgamate, and even space exists also from dispersion of *qi*. Expanding from Zhang's model, Zhu Xi 朱熹 (1130–1200) developed his famous theory explaining the relationship between *qi* and *li* 理 (principles). Zhu posits that all things in the cosmos share *qi* and *li*. There must be *li*, or the core principles, that result in the consistent patterns that transcend across dimensions. But there must also be *qi* to serve as the physical matter from which the patterns would actually "materialize." The inherent principles in the cosmos dictate the actual form of any given being; the *qi* matter also cannot manifest into actual form without the principles. Nothing in the cosmos can exist unless there is both *li* and *qi*. Zhu states simply: "Humans exist because *li* and *qi* came together."[22]

Precisely because *qi* and *li* are essential for existence and universal in all things, it is then crucial to understand what those principles might be. The shared principles warrant that if we know the principles within one thing, we would know the principles in all things in the world and all aspects of human life. To Zhu, *li* is the inherent patterns of *Dao*, which precedes the physical existence that manifests through *qi*. Therefore, for humans to truly understand *Dao*, one must observe the patterns in nature and extrapolate the principles that govern these shared patterns. For most effective understanding of these shared principles, Zhu believes that one's mind must be fully present and alert. He promotes quiet sitting (*jingzuo* 靜坐) and meditation (*chan* 禪) to cultivate that state of absolute attentiveness and reverence (*jing* 敬). Besides rigorous mental discipline, there is a certain physical attitude involved in the cultivation: "The head should be upright, the eyes looking straight ahead, the feet steady, the hands respectful, the mouth quiet and composed, the bearing solemn—these are all aspects of inner mental attentiveness."[23]

The physical component of mental cultivation exemplifies the classical Chinese understanding of mind as part of the physical body, and spirit as inseparable from the physical form. The spirit aspect of a person is therefore not just part of the physical reality of human existence. It is considered an alternate form of *qi* that is consistent with the physical body, and tangible through its correspondence with the physical body. In modern day TCM, Chinese ethnic practitioners refer to the physically tangible and observable aspects of *qi* to validate and legitimize their clinical practices.

SENSING THE *QI*

Regardless of individual understandings and positions on the issue of "spiritual," every TCM practitioner I have talked to is able and willing to talk to me about how important *qi* is to their clinical practices. Dr. Yuan is one of many Chinese ethnic practitioners who insists that TCM should be first understood as a medicine, and as a science:

> This is medicine and it is scientific. My personal feeling is that [traditional Chinese medicine] is not something fraudulent, so [people] should not make it all mysterious (*xuan* 玄), like some cultish folks (*shengun* 神棍) do. Even if there are extrasensory abilities (*teyi gongneng* 特異功能), those are hard to measure [scientifically]. The natural world as a whole has many things that we do not understand. *Qigong* is not something I understand or have any interest in. To me, that is mysterious.

Jason also frames traditional Chinese medicine first and foremost as scientific:

> The Chinese understanding of Chinese medicine is very scientific (*kexue* 科學). Good *zhongyi*[24] all think that Chinese medicine is scientific. Those who don't understand Chinese medicine or those who talk nonsense... when *zhongyi* gets to the US it changes flavor, just like Chinese food comes to the US and the flavor changes... [it becomes] American-Chinese, tastes not the same. A lot of American folks think that Chinese

medicine is miraculous (*shen* 神), [as in] *shenxian* 神仙 (gods or deities) . . . and don't talk about things like *qi* more scientifically. *Zhongyi* talk about *qi*, but it's in fact a type of [physiological] pushing force of the heart. Or heat, light, and energy . . . things that can be detected physically. The kind of *qi* that [the Americans] talk about talks about nothing at all (*yanzhi wuwu* 言之無物). Truly outstanding *zhongyishi*[25] must be very scientific.

When asked what he means by "scientific," Jason explains:

> *Kexue* is when things can be studied and experimented (*yanjiu* 研究), tangible, with physical forms (*xingxiang* 形象), subjective, can be touched. Religion (*zongjiao*) you can't touch physically. The sensation of *qi* (*qigan* 氣感) is scientific.

To Jason, Science is physical, tangible, and observable, while religion is *not* physical, tangible, or observable. In other words, to him, science and religion are polar opposites. He goes on to expand on how *qi* not only exists but can be detected scientifically:

> The sensation of *qi* can be detected [scientifically]. Nowadays some exams, like for women's breasts they do mammogram, they use special infrared cameras to make temperature mapping. That you can't [normally] see, right? But when you take a picture like that, if you find a spot that gives more heat, then there is where a cyst it. That is *qi*. Chinese medicine talks about the stagnation of *qi* and conglomeration of phlegm (*qizhi tanyu* 氣滯痰淤) or the stagnation of *qi* and conglomeration of blood (*qizhi xueyu* 氣滯血淤), the *qi* is blocked there, and if it's blocked there for long, [the spot] warms up. After it warms up, there will be inflammations, and there will be [abnormal] growth. Then when a mammogram is taken, the growth will show. Mammogram won't catch a growth unless it's already pretty big, but if there is slight inflammation, that heat from the inflammation is already concentrated at that spot, and it will show up on the temperature map. From the perspective of Western medicine, what is detected is a structure, an actual material mass is formed.

The two practitioners' defensive tones and repeated assertions that TCM is "scientific" reflect a collective struggle deeply embedded in the Chinese cultural identity. For more than a century, China's reactions against the invasions of, oppressions by, and competitions with the Western powers had become an obsession toward becoming a modern nation. The majority of Chinese elites had resented the baggage of the Confucian system and folk religious cults, deeming them as hindrances to the growth of the nation; they also criticized the Chinese tradition for lacking the logics of Western philosophy and the rigor of Western science, which to them explains why the Western nations had the upper hand in global economy and power dynamics. Therefore, the contrast between scientific and religious is not so much about what is science and what is religion, but rather, what is considered modern, advanced, more effective, and thus superior, versus what would be otherwise—the primitive, backward, less effective, and therefore inferior. Often, the Chinese immigrant TCM practitioners still feel the need to validate TCM as a modern, advanced medical system by showing, or at least by claiming, that it is scientific.

Nonetheless, as practitioners talk more about TCM's own theoretical paradigm, the concept of *qi* becomes central. Dr. Yuan explains:

> In relation to acupuncture, Chinese medicine talks about *qi*, and to use external *qi* to treat illness, I think that is possible. When we do acupuncture, we can sometimes sense (vibrate with or in empathetic resonance with; *ganying* 感應[26]) the external *qi*. Like the sensation in the hand when [the needle] *deqi*, we can sense it after some practice. Some other [forms] of *qi* cannot be sensed. That's my personal feeling.

Jason also describes how TCM uses early detection of the *qi* stagnation or even prevention of illnesses:

> *Zhongyi* sometimes take a look and know, oh you have a problem. Western doctors need to get more tests done, when there is an image to prove then they can say they know. That's already too late. So Chinese medicine talks about *wang wen wen qie* 望聞問切 [look, listen, ask, and determine], and we say "If you can know by just looking, that is *shen* 神" (wang-er zhizhi weizhi shen 望而知之謂之神). Knowing by a general look, that can be done by very experienced doctors. Experience is also science. For Western medicine, some people appear to be healthy but are not truly healthy. Things that Western medicine talk about, very often when [illness] is discovered, it is already too late.

The character 神 *shen*, besides being the "spirit" aspect of the *jing-qi-shen* trio, has connotations across different dimensions. As an adjective, it describes things being so incredible that it becomes miraculous, as in *shenqi* 神奇. While Jason quotes the saying to emphasize the power of experience, another common definition of the character 神, especially when it is used as a noun, is that of a deity or a god. The ambiguity of grammar in classical Chinese easily renders the saying with two possible interpretations: 1) If you can know by just looking, that is incredibly skillful; or 2) If you can know by just looking, you are essentially at the level of knowing as a god. And the two interpretations do not necessarily conflict with each other; the saying can be inclusive of both interpretations. On the other hand, the fuzzy inclusion of *qi* into the physical by the virtue of its tangibility (it can be sensed and scientifically observed) also effectively brings the "mysterious" into the legitimate realm.

Clinically, the concept of *deqi*, a unique sensation induced by the insertion of a needle into an acupuncture point that indicates successful positioning and flow of *qi*, is very important in the practice of acupuncture.[27] Dr. Yuan gives a succinct and concise description of *deqi*:

> There are two aspects to *deqi*: one is the patient's sensation, and also the sensation by the one who applies [the needle]. Clinically this is not so hard, when you [sense] *deqi* then you tell the patient that the needle has achieved *deqi*. *Deqi* has to do with human anatomy and the sensation under the needle. With practice, one can start to feel that somewhere under the needle [along the path of insertion] it gets heavier. At first the resistance is less, but at a certain point it gets tighter. After the needle is inserted, there are also reactions like redness and heat [on the skin]. There are phenomena that are subjective.

From the healer's perspective, there are also visible and even tactile signs of *deqi*. Meilun describes:

> [The practitioner] would be able to feel a difference in the needle. For example, when you *deqi*, the *qi* is unblocked. Some patients have lower back pain, back pain, I acupuncture points on the back. After the needles go in the patient is there, face down, with nothing covering her. Or I might use the infrared lamp over her lower back section. Then what happens? The patient's back of the heels and the tendons start to heat up, and become warmer to the touch than any other part of the body. I've opened up the bladder meridian. After I take the needles off, I let the patient get up to touch the spots, or have another patient come touch the backs of the heels. There was nothing covering her, and other parts of the legs are cooler, only the backs of the heels are warmer. I can even see that it gets a little redder. There are such phenomena, so how do you explain that? That is *qi*. But what is *qi*? There are many people studying and researching that. Chinese have also researched for many years, but there is yet to be a conclusion.

Rather than providing an intellectual conclusion for the patients, most of the TCM practitioners I talked to and observed actually guide their patients to explore the Chinese understanding of human through the articulations of bodily sensations—the very subtle sensations that are only observable and identifiable after some training in self-inspection. Some of these sensations are more commonly identified in the American culture, such as numbness, soreness, tenderness, and pain. Other sensations, such as hot and cold (not in terms of temperature but the subjective sensation), or dry and damp (there are concrete physical signs to these conditions, but also specific sensations attached to them) are not categories that have ready equivalents in the mainstream American culture.

The sensation of *qi* is, above all, most foreign to American culture. What does a thing feel like if you never knew it existed? Granted, although the concept of *qi* is widely understood in Chinese societies and the character profusely used in the Chinese language, not everyone who is immersed in Chinese culture has necessarily experienced or known the sensation of *qi* on and in his or her body. Precisely because *qi* is invisible and not tangible to the uninitiated, most people who can sense *qi* were trained into sensing it. Those who are ambivalent toward the claim that the invisible *qi* exists can easily argue that the *qi* sensation is a phenomenon of group imagination or fantasy. Conversely, if we assume that *qi* is part of the human body, just like skin, bones, muscles, and blood, then there is no reason why we cannot try to understand the training of *qi* sensation—or in the case of *qigong* and other *qi* cultivations, *qi* control—along the same lines as training muscles to drastically increase one's strength. Furthermore, there have now been several scientific research reports on how the existence and movements of *qi* can be proven by changes in electrical currents along where the meridians are supposed to be on the body.[28] The findings are consistent with the common analogy of the sensation with *qi*, with shots of electrical currents through meridians, especially when needles are inserted in certain acupuncture points or when *qi* infusion is performed along the meridians.

The bodily sensations take training to understand, and some sensations also serve as markers for illnesses. For example, plum pit *qi*, or *meihe qi* 梅核氣, is a sensation that feels like a small solid mass, or something that feels like a small plum's pit, is stuck in one's throat. The sensation makes one constantly want to clear the throat, and indicates accumulation of phlegm in the throat that stems from emotional causes. Although there are other aspects of the standard diagnoses[29] that can help the practitioner determine a patient's physical condition, accurate understanding of these categories of sensations is helpful, if not crucial, in properly applying the knowledge of traditional Chinese medicine in clinical practice. Not only do the practitioners have to be familiar with these sensations; without the shared cultural knowledge of these sensations being common sense, practitioners also have to train their patients to notice and articulate these sensations.

Sensations—something that we often take for granted yet is profoundly indicative of our existence—are also highly subjective. Furthermore, the process of a previously unlabeled and thus mostly unnoticed sensation to suddenly take on a name and meaning can be conceptually transformational and may even seem magical. The magical quality of these newly identified sensations is even more pronounced when they are taken as completely natural, universal, and self-explanatory.

Qi, something that is invisible but can be sensed after some training, is believed to be part of the physical world and its existence self-explanatory. As part of their cultural knowledge, Chinese ethnic practitioners see *qi* as the basic element that makes up all things in the world and the foundation for all bodily functions. Therefore, human sensations in the Chinese context have historically been defined with the existence of *qi* as one basic reference point. When TCM crossed a cultural boundary into mainstream America, the existing American culture did not have a shared understanding of the existence or the sensation of *qi*. However, even when the explanations with *qi* as an element seem confusing, the efficacy of the TCM treatments makes the explanation more believable, although sometimes with a grain of salt. Before one is initiated into the *qi* sensation, one must first "believe" in its existence in order for the explanations to be valid. Then even when one is aware of the *qi* sensation, the subjectivity of sensations still leaves many to wonder whether it is really a physical sensation and not a spiritual experience.

CORRESPONDENCE BETWEEN LAYERS OF EXISTENCE

In the TCM theoretical paradigm, the correspondence between emotions and the physical body is direct and concrete. By sharing the categories of the five elements, each major emotion is tied to a meridian, which reflects the energetic functions and processes of one *yin* organ (*zang* 臟) and one *yang* organ (*fu* 腑). Furthermore, also by categorization under the five elements, there are body parts, sensations, and qualities of a person's appearance that are related to each emotion.

The somatic implication of Table 11.1 is that emotional conditions, even if not expressed directly, have observable physical functions, locations, and signs that are understood to be connected to the emotions. And because the correspondence is based on the resonance of having the characteristics of the same elemental category, emotional problems can be observed through bodily signs such as the smell of the patient's breath, and the color of her countenance. Treating or improving the condition of any of the corresponding attributes can have positive effects on the emotion.

For example, if a patient has a red tint in her countenance, and even has a burnt smell in her breath, that is a sign that she may have some imbalance or even disease in her heart and small intestine meridians. It is possible that the health of her tongue and the blood vessels in her body are already affected as well. She may already notice feeling angry and

Table 11.1.

Emotion	Anger	Elation	Melancholy	Grief	Fear
Element	Wood	Fire	Earth	Metal	Water
Yin Organ	Liver	Heart	Spleen	Lungs	Kidney
Yang Organ	Gall Bladder	Small Intestine	Stomach	Large Intestine	Bladder
Orifice	Eyes	Tongue	Mouth	Nose	Ears
Tissue	Tendons	Blood Vessels	Flesh	Skin	Bones
Smell	Goatish	Burnt	Fragrant	Fishy	Rotten
Color Tint of Countenance	Blue-green	Red	Yellow	White	Black

generally getting more short-tempered. If her physical condition deteriorates, her temper might also get worse. Likewise, if she does not control her temper, her physical condition might worsen. Therefore, clinical treatment can focus on treating her physical condition, and as the heart and small intestines meridians are unblocked and functions are properly restored, her temper might improve. Also, if she consciously tries to control her temper, the treatments for her heart and small-intestine conditions might be even more effective. By resonance, there is actual somatic basis for emotions; treating and managing one or more of the corresponding attributes only improves the general conditions of all of them. The healing is holistic because corresponding layers are actually being treated all at the same time.

This synchronized, resonating process is called *ganying*, variously translated by Western academics as stimulus-response, sympathetic resonance,[30] impulse and response,[31] or response and retribution.[32] In a most general, naturalistic way of understanding the process, *ganying* is

> a mode of seemingly spontaneous response (although not in the sense of "uncaused") natural in a universe conceived holistically in terms of pattern and interdependent order. Resonance as the mechanism through which categorically related yet spatially distant phenomena interact. . . . Objects belonging to the same category or class spontaneously resonate with each other just as do two identical tuned strings on a pair of zithers.[33]

Another interpretation touches upon the juxtaposition between human and nature on different levels:

> [*Ganying*] means that nothing happens without an impact on or a connection to everything else. All is closely interrelated not only by causes but also synchronously, i.e., events are not seen following each other in the same places at the same time. In other words, according to this view, whenever something happens in one plane of existence, there is a more or less immediate echo on all the others. Earthquakes, for example, or changes in the course of the planet, have their matching events in human society and in people's bodies. And conversely, political events are mirrored in natural and planetary movements or disasters.[34]

The concept of *ganying* provides a non-hierarchical framework for understanding why the articulation of somatic sensation is crucial in TCM. One's body, being the closest observable aspect of existence that is also connected to all other aspects of existence by the shared material of *qi* and shared patterns of *yinyang* and the five elements, is an ideal vantage point for understanding not only what is in the body, but also what is in the human society and in nature. Due to this recognition of interconnectedness, discomfort, imbalance, and dysfunctions of the physical body are inevitably related to the emotional and spiritual well-being of the person as well. Unlike the Western psychiatric model where the somatized conditions are seen as uni-directionally transferring the unarticulated emotional and psychological distress onto the physical body, the *ganying* model posits that when one of the corresponding layers, regardless of which one, exhibits imbalance or illness, all layers are inevitably affected, and treatment can then be applied on any layer to heal all layers. Better yet, treatments on multiple layers simultaneously will expedite the healing of the underlying energetic patterns and dynamics that somehow went askew.

SPIRITUAL: THE REFINEMENT OF *QI*

In the context of the TCM clinics in the Bay Area, we see how crucial the physical sensations of *qi* and observable signs of *deqi* are, not only to give credibility to the healers and the healing modalities, but also to provide physical basis for the *qi*-oriented theoretical model behind the clinical practices. The patients are trained to articulate their somatic sensations so that they can provide valuable insights for their own bodily conditions, and feedback on the effectiveness of the treatments they receive. This is the level of application of the knowledge of *qi* that most TCM practitioners aim for. Although some practitioners incorporate other types of spiritual assistance in their clinical practices, by no means do I suggest that the practitioners collectively attempt to preach or promote a systematic spirituality.

However, the experiential understanding of *qi* through sensations in the physical body conceptually expands the boundary of the human body. The effect of the conceptual paradigm is most apparent on patients who visit clinics regularly for long-term health maintenance. With the articulation of and discourse on *qi* sensations, practitioners help the patients tap into all manifestations of *qi*. By prescribing herbs and food with specific elemental and medicinal qualities, and by incorporating non-TCM supplements in the treatment plans, the practitioners help the patients cultivate the *jing*, or the nourishing essence, of their body. Administering acupuncture on the patients is a way to unblock and manage the *qi* in the meridians. Those practitioners who do *qi*-infusion clinically and promote and teach *qigong* practices, are also actively helping their patients cultivate—not only gather and store, but also purify—the *qi*. At times the *shen* (spirit) dimension is also touched upon. Herbs and acupuncture can be administered to calm the spirit, with the goal of promoting less turbulence in the general condition of *qi* in the patient's body. It is also understood that by correspondence, balancing the *yinyang* and the five elements in the physical body means that one's emotional and mental states are going to resonate and become more balanced as well.

Therefore, the "spiritual" in TCM healing also lies in the process of that progression from the more materialistic *jing*, to the cultivation of *qi*, and in that constant refinement of *qi*. If *shen* is indeed the purest, finest form of *qi*, then by becoming more balanced, more refined, and healthier, one becomes spiritual as well.

NOTES

1. See Paul Steven Sangren, *History and Magical Power in a Chinese Community* (Stanford: Stanford University Press, 1987), 264.
2. See Xingzhong Yao, *An Introduction to Confucianism* (New York: Cambridge University Press, 2000), 91. Yao uses the term mainly in conjunction and contrast with *li* 理, the metaphysical principle, in the Neo-Confucian discourse on the relationship between *qi* and *li*.
3. See Daniel Gardner, *Learning to Be a Sage: Selections from the Conversations of Master Chu, Arranged Topically* (Berkeley: University of California Press, 1990), 50–51. Gardner uses this translation to encompass the psychological and mental aspect of *qi* in the scheme of Neo-Confucian education and cultivation.
4. Lunyu, chapter 7, "Shu-er 述而": 子不語怪力亂神。
5. See Confucius and Arthur Waley, *The Analects of Confucius* (New York: Vintage Books, 1989), 127.
6. See Confucius and Dim Cheuk Lau, *The Analects* (Harmondsworth; New York: Penguin Books, 1979), 88.
7. See James Legge, *Confucian Analects* (Whitefish, MT: Kessinger Publishing, 2004), 52.
8. Guanzi, "Shuyan 樞言": 有氣則生，無氣則死，生者以其氣。得之必生，失者必死者，何也？唯氣。
9. Zhuangzi, chapter 22 "Zhibeiyou 知北遊": 人之生，氣之聚也。聚則為生，散則為死。
10. Daodejing: 陰陽陶冶萬物，皆乘一氣而生。
11. Zhuangzi, chapter 18, "Zhile 至樂": 氣變而有形，形變而有生。
12. Huangdi Neijing Suwen, chapter 39, "Jutong Lun 舉痛論": 余知百病生於氣也，怒則氣上，喜則氣緩，悲則氣消，恐則氣下，寒則氣收，炅則氣泄，驚則氣亂，勞則氣耗，思則氣結。
13. Xin 心 is often translated as the heart, but in Chinese culture the term encompasses both the physiological organ of the heart, and many qualities of the mind. *Xin* in a person not only thinks logically but also feels emotionally.
14. Liezi, chapter 2, "Huangdi 黃帝": 而後眼如耳，耳如鼻，鼻如口，無不同也。心凝形釋，骨肉都融。
15. See Shigeru Ishida, "Looking at the Characteristics of Ancient Chinese View of the Body through the Knowledge of the Development Process of the Body (You Shenti Shengcheng Guocheng De Renshi Laikan Zhongguo Gudai Shentiguan De Tezhi 由身體生成過程的認識來看中國古代身體觀的特質)," in *Qi Theories and Conception of the Body in Ancient Chinese Thoughts (Zhongguo Gudai Sixiang Zhong De Qilun Ju Shentiguan 中國古代思想中的氣論及身體觀*, ed. Ru-Bin Yang 楊儒賓 (Taipei: Juliu Publishing, 1993), 185–86.
16. See Fuchen Hu, "The Tri-Level Xing, Qi, Shen Structured Conception of the Body in Daoist Thoughts and Daoist Religion (Daojia He Daojiao Xing Qi Shen Sanchong Jiegou De Rentiguan 道家和道教形，氣，神三重結構的人體觀)," in *Qi Theories and Conception of the Body in Ancient Chinese Thoughts (Zhongguo Gudai Sixiang Zhong De Qilun Ju Shentiguan 中國古代思想中的氣論及身體觀)*, ed. Ru-Bin Yang (Taipei: Juliu Publishing, 1993), 173.
17. Baopuzi, "Zhili 至理": 身勞則神散，氣竭則命終。
18. Hu, "The Tri-Level Xing, Qi, Shen Structured Conception of the Body in Daoist Thoughts and Daoist Religion (Daojia He Daojiao Xing Qi Shen Sanchong Jiegou De Rentiguan 道家和道教形，氣，神三重結構的人體觀)," 173.

19. Zhonghe ji, chapter 2, 煉精化氣，煉氣化神，煉神還虛。
20. Huainanzi, chapter 7, "Jingshen Xun精神訓": 夫精神者，所受於天也；而形體者，所稟於地也。故頭之圓也象天，足之方也象地。天有四時、五行、九解、三百六十六日，人亦有四支、五藏、九竅、三百六十六節。天有風雨寒暑，人亦有取與喜怒。
21. Lunheng, chapter 62, "Lunsi 論死": 氣之生人，猶水之為冰也。水凝為冰，氣凝為人；冰釋為水，人死復神。其名為神也，猶冰釋更名水也。
22. Zhuzi Yulei 朱子語類, chapter 4, 人之所以生，理與氣合而已。
23. Daniel Gardner, *Chu Hsi: Learning to Be a Sage*, 172. Gardner's translation of Zhu Xi's original passage.
24. Please see a discussion of the term *zhongyi* 中醫 (traditional Chinese doctors) in the introductory chapter.
25. *Zhongyishi* 中醫師 is synonymous to *zhongyi*. Please also see the introductory chapter.
26. There will be more on this concept later in this chapter. For a historical analysis of the term within the Chinese religious context, see Robert H. Sharf, *Coming to Terms with Chinese Buddhism: A Reading of the Treasure Store Treatise* (Honolulu: University of Hawai'i Press, 2002), 82–88.
27. Several recent quantitative and qualitative researches have been conducted on the experiences, characteristics, and explanations of *deqi*. See J. Kong et al., "Acupuncture De Qi, from Qualitative History to Quantitative Measurement," *Journal of Alternative and Complementary Medicine* 13, no. 10 (2007): 1059-1070; H. MacPherson and A. Asghar, "Acupuncture Needle Sensations Associated with De Qi: A Classification Based on Experts' Ratings," *Journal of Alternative and Complementary Medicine* 12, no. 7 (2006): 633–37; J. J. Mao et al., "De Qi: Chinese Acupuncture Patients' Experiences and Beliefs Regarding Acupuncture Needling Sensation—an Exploratory Survey," *Acupuncture Medicine* 25, no. 4 (2007): 158–65; K.K. Hui et al., "Characterization of The 'Deqi' Response in Acupuncture," *BMC Complementary Alternative Medicine* 7, no. 33 (2007) http://www.biomedcentral.com/content/pdf/1472-6882-7-33.pdf (accessed April 7, 2010).
28. See A.C. Ahn and others, "Electrical Properties of Acupuncture Points and Meridians: A Systematic Review," *Bioelectromagnetics* 29, no. 4 (2008): 245–56.
29. Standard TCM diagnosis has four components: *wang*望 (to look or observe the color and appearance of face, tongue, whites of the eyes, and so on), *wen*聞 (to listen to the sound of breathing and coughs, and to smell the odor of breath coming out of the body of the patient), *wen*問 (to ask patients questions on background of the complaint and other subjective feelings and observations), and *qie*切 (to check pulse on both wrists).
30. See Sharf, *Coming to Terms with Chinese Buddhism: A Reading of the Treasure Store Treatise*.
31. Kohn, *Daoism and Chinese Culture*, 45.
32. See introduction by D. T. Suzuki to his translation of Treatise on Response & Retribution 太上感應經: Laozi, D. T. Suzuki, and Paul Carus, *Treatise on Response and Retribution* (La Salle, IL: Open Court Publishing, 1973). Because the text is a Daoist treatise, the term "retribution" encompasses the moral dimension in the interaction between humans and the divine.
33. Sharf, *Coming to Terms with Chinese Buddhism: A Reading of the Treasure Store Treatise*, 83.
34. Kohn, *Daoism and Chinese Culture*, 45.

TWELVE
Ideal Body and Concept of Health

According to the World Health Organization (WHO), health is defined as "a state of complete physical, mental and social well-being and not merely the absence of disease or infirmity."[1] The National Institute of Health (NIH) articulates health in close conjunction with wellness, lifestyle, and disease prevention.[2] These officially established definitions of health are intentionally broad, and provide much space for interpretation.

Many experienced TCM practitioners recognize that the market advantage of traditional Chinese medicine is in providing holistic care that covers physical, emotional, and even spiritual healing. The TCM system assumes that different dimensions of human existence correspond and resonate with one another. Consequently, physical modalities can be used to treat emotional and spiritual conditions. Alternatively, physical conditions can also benefit from an improved state of emotional and spiritual balance.

Medical acupuncturist Leon Hammer identifies the directional difference between the biomedical and TCM approaches toward healing. He observes that the Western medical model seeks to measure the physical aspects of disease to the very minute level, which is limited: "Preventative medicine in the West is, at best, an early warning system of an already existing morphological, identifiable lesion."[3] Furthermore, the biomedical model "works from the serious disease and death-end of the spectrum" toward a healthier state of being, which "has thus far proven to be an expensive and futile exercise in the quest of early diagnosis and prevention."[4]

On the other hand, the Chinese medical model works "from the health-end of the spectrum," where "any act by man or nature which interferes with the quantity, circulation, or rhythmic balance of the life force, or energy, will lead in the direction of disease and toward the death end of the spectrum."[5] In other words, TCM strives for maintaining an ultimate balance, and preventive measures start with the slightest signs of deviation from that state of balance. Since *qi* is the basic life force and material of the physical body in the TCM framework, "physiology" includes more than just what is physical. This explains why TCM considers somatized symptoms as real physical disease. The recognition of an energetic alteration as the earliest sign of disorder allows for prevention of disease before it progresses to the disease of the cellular, physical body.

In this chapter, we will explore how TCM practitioners help their patients strive for health, which is defined by the maintenance of balance. I will first investigate the Chinese classical and cultural model for the ideal states of the body, and how "balance" is defined clinically based on the model. In the TCM clinics, we will see how cross-cultural, social, and environmental discourses in the Californian context also contribute to the definition of health. Beyond physical and energetic balance, TCM in the American context also extend the concept of health to include the understanding of interconnectedness between humans and nature, and between people in a shared space and in a community.

MODEL FOR IDEAL STATE OF BODY

In the TCM clinics in the Bay Area that I have visited and observed, besides the short-term goal of addressing the obvious symptoms that brought the patient to the clinic in the first place, there are often also longer-term goals that the practitioners hope to achieve—there is an ideal state of the body that is considered healthy. Of course, the patients do not all return for more treatments after the main clinical complaint is taken care of, but many do, and they often become the stable patient base that sustain the clinics. TCM practitioners and textual resources point to three important conditions that contribute to the state of health: 1) the *qi* in the meridians of the body flows unobstructed, smoothly, and evenly like well-managed rivers; 2) the balance within the body—between the functional organ systems and between different aspects of human existence—first restored and hopefully maintained; 3) the patient has abundant supply of beneficial *qi* to supply for the proper functioning of the body, and ideally is connected to the cosmic *qi* source through self-cultivation, contact with nature, or the help of *qi*-abundant practitioners.

Managing and Balancing the System

In the Chinese language, diseases are "managed" rather than just treated. The character *zhi* 治 in the compound word *zhibing* 治病, an equivalent of treating illness, literally means "to manage." A common compound word *zhili* 治理, meaning to manage and to put into order, is used across medical healing, political governing, and prevention of floods from river overflow. Incidentally, Chinese cultivation and medical classics analogize the human body both to a political system and a water system. According to the understanding of shared principles across microcosm and macrocosm, the human body, a governing hierarchy, and the natural waterways all have corresponding features that can be juxtaposed, and share the same patterns that can be managed with strategies sharing the same core principles.

The *Huangting jing* 黃庭經 (The Scriptures of the Yellow Court) is a central text in the Shangqing 上清 (Highest Clarity) school of Daoism. Part of the text, "The Outer Radiance Scripture of the Yellow Court" (Huangting waijing jing 黃庭外景經) is often attributed to the founder of the Shangqing school, Wei Huacun 魏華存 (252–334), with the other two parts added later to complement. These inner cultivation texts are consistent with providing a detailed interior vision of the human body as chambers and halls where gods reside and rule. The central tenet of the Yellow Court scriptures is that inside each compartment, inside the head, at every organ, and in every joint of the body, there resides a god. Here is how *The Inner Radiance Scripture of the Yellow Court* (Huangting neijing jing 黃庭內景經) lists the gods in the head, also known as the Niwan 泥丸 Palace, and describes how they govern:

> The god of hair, Canghua, is also called Taiyuan. The god of brain, Jinggan, is also called Niwan. The god of eyes, Mingshang, is also called Yingxuan. The god of nose, Yugong, is also called Lingjian. The god of ears, Kongcian, is also called Youtian. The god of tongue, Tongming, is also called Zhenglun. The god of teeth, Efeng, is also called Luoqian. Niwan is the leader of the Niwan Palace. There are also nine true spirits in the palace (who report to the head of the palace) each with their own chamber, [each chamber] about one inch in size. They share a purple robe made from luxurious fabric. Thinking about any one of these gods will bring longevity. They don't all just live in the brain, but are seated in order and face outward, and correspond to each other.[6]

Like local officials governing a nation, the gods in the human body govern different parts of the body with the same basic principles of political governance. As Daoists were usually not expert political advisors like the Confucians, the image of a political hierarchy in the body in this Daoist description is more akin to the hierarchy of the celestial officials of the Daoist pantheon, which in turn mirrored the hierarchy of the imperial government.

The Chinese medical classic *Huangdi Neijing Lingshu* 黃帝內經靈樞 (The Yellow Emperor's Inner Classic: Spiritual Pivot) superimposes the human body with natural landscapes:

> The five *yin* organs, six *yang* organs, and the twelve meridians—they are all supported externally from the water source, and managed internally. They connect to each other outside and inside, like a ring without end. This is the same with the human meridians. The heaven above is *yang*, and the earth below is *yin*; above the waist is the heaven, and below the waist is earth. Therefore, the location north of "the water of the sea" (stomach) is called *Yin*. The location north of "the lake" (spleen) is called "*Yin* in the *Yin*." The location of the Zhang River (pericardium) is called *Yang*. The region north of the "water of the stream" (lung) to the water of the Zhang River is called "*Yin* in the *Yang*." The region south of the water of Luo River (triple warmer) to the water of the stream is called "*Yang* in the *Yang*." These are examples illustrated with parts of the waters in certain locations, and it is the principle of the correspondence between human and the cosmos.[7]

In this model, the rivers in the body share the same core characteristics as rivers in nature. Therefore, principles for "managing" the rivers in nature can be applied when a healer strategizes her treatment plans.

George, our Bay Area expert on Chinese medical classics, demonstrates the classical irrigation model through the discussion on diabetes:

> In Chinese medicine, meridians are rivers. In the human body there are four seas, the brain, bones, blood, and *qi*; four seas. The four seas are connected by the blood vessels in the body, and the meridians are rivers. In these rivers, cholesterol corresponds with the Earth phase. Sugar is sweet, among the five elements, the taste that corresponds with Earth is sweetness. Metal corresponds with spiciness, Fire corresponds with bitterness, Wood corresponds with sourness, and Water corresponds with saltiness. Fatty things and muscles are related to the spleen, and spleen corresponds with Earth. When more of these [Earthy] things accumulate inside the blood vessels, like eating too greasy, these accumulate, it's like a lot of soil in water, like the Yellow River [in China]. Yellow River is in a condition of high cholesterol. Why high cholesterol? The river bed gets higher and higher. How high? It's now more than twenty meters higher than the cities by the river. Once the levees break, think about it, the cities must be flooded. But how did the river bed get so high? Because the river bed has a lot of soil . . . soil is Earth, and it is just like the lipid and blood sugar inside blood vessels. How does TCM treat that? Western medicine treats high blood pressure by reducing the pressure: when there is a lot of blood, it exerts more pressure on the blood vessels, so they use diuretics. Why use diuretics? Because they want to reduce the volume of the blood. Just like nowadays, when the Yellow River is treated, they drain out the water in it by branching it out.

He then transitions seamlessly into designing a treatment plan based on balancing the five elements:

> That is one way, but not the best way, and not a way to treat the root of the problem, just treating the symptoms. So what is the way to treat the

Ideal Body and Concept of Health 193

root problem? At least we need to take away some of that soil, that is the train of thought toward treating the root problem, removing the Earth. How do you remove the Earth? You can just dig, but there is more soil continuously coming down from upstream, and after you dig some, more soil comes along. The source of the problem is whether there are trees upstream. If there are trees and they are all green, the tree roots stabilize the soil [by holding on to soil] and there won't be lost soil [going downstream]. Trees are woods, and liver corresponds with Wood [element], so the root problem of diabetes is in the liver. If the liver is taken care of, [the person] is happy, with nothing to stress over and nothing to worry about, then there is no diabetes or high blood pressure.[8]

Not all TCM practitioners incorporate the five elements theory into their clinical treatment, but all would emphasize the importance of balance, be that balance between *yang* and *yin*, hot and cold, surplus and deficiency, or just a sense of moderation. Dr. Zhang (see chapter 7), who prescribes herbal tonics and soup recipes to her patients, insists that most of her San Francisco patients need to abstain from cold food, such as raw, iced food, most fruits, and vegetables that have a bitter taste. She prescribes a lot of warming, hot food such as ginger, dried *longan* fruits, cinnamon, pepper, sesame oil, and toasted beans and nuts. The "hot" and "cold" refer to not only the actual temperature of the food, but more importantly, the natural effects of the food on the human body when it is consumed. She believes the chilling *qi* that is characteristic of San Francisco, and certain habits in the modern lifestyle ("Ice water is for people who wish to get sick quickly," says Dr. Zhang) make her patients too cold, which not only slows metabolism, but also contributes to excess accumulation of phlegm, stagnant *qi* in the meridians, and eventually even abnormal growths inside the body. Her prescriptions aim to warm the body systematically so that it would start functioning properly by itself. "Hot is *yang* and cold is *yin*," she explains, "if we can balance the hot and cold properly, that is to balance the *yin* and *yang* too."

Crystal (see chapter 2), who uses mostly acupuncture, expressed a similar approach to balancing the *yin* and *yang* during our interview. In the middle of our conversation, she suddenly asked me to stick out my tongue so that she could take a better look at it, a request that I am actually familiar with, growing up in a medical family and with an acupuncturist mother. Crystal took a closer look at my tongue, and exclaimed, "You are too cold, and deficient in *qi*! Even if you don't do anything else, please at least drink lots of hot ginger water to keep warm!"

Filling Up with Qi

In a public lecture in 2008, sinologist and historian of Chinese medicine Paul Unschuld shared a cross-cultural shift he observed in the TCM theoretical paradigm in the United States: Historically a mainly agrarian culture, Chinese traditionally analogizes human bodily functions with water irrigations and rivers. On the other hand, non-Chinese American TCM practitioners and patients, first introduced to TCM during an era of energy crisis, understand human mechanisms through the analogy of energy, where the human body is seen as something like a battery.[9]

In the Bay Area, where China-trained practitioners and educators are numerous and active, I observed a coexistence and sometimes a mixture of both paradigms. The irrigation model, as described in the previous section, is exemplified as meridians being channels for *qi* that must be kept unblocked. Blockage in the meridians is a major cause for imbalance, pain, and illness. The quality of *qi* flow is also important. Practitioners who do pulse diagnosis can feel the very subtle quality of the *qi* flow in each of the meridians—healthy pulses exhibit *qi* flow in the meridians with appropriate pace, fullness, clarity, depth, and so on.

A Caucasian American clinical training instructor in the TCM school explains how she determines her treatment plan depending on the time of the day:

> If the patients come in earlier in the day, then I would sometimes put a needle in to boost the energy, that way they will be energized for the rest of the day. But if the patients come at the end of the day, then I would do a calming needle so that they can go home, relax, and have a good night's sleep.[10]

This is indeed analogizing the human body as a battery, where one would want to charge it up for an active day, or drain it down for a restful night. Using needles, *qigong*, and other cultivation and healing methods, the TCM practitioners help their patients connect to the power sources that provide *qi*, very much as electronics are connected to power outlets and batteries to function.

The battery paradigm, I argue, is only a partial innovation. The analogy to a battery, which is a modern invention, and the concerns of the energy crisis, are indeed products of the Western modernized world. However, the concept of filling the physical body with *qi* to improve the functioning of the whole person has classical sources. Huainanzi promotes filling and storing the gut with *qi*:

> When the blood and *qi* can be contained within the five inner organs (Liver, Heart, Spleen, Stomach, and Kidney) and not leak, then the chest and abdomen would become full, and appetite for food will decrease. Then the ears and eyes are clear, and one sees and hears well ... and that is clarity. When the spirit (jingshen) is vibrant and the vital

force (qi) is not scattered, then [the body] is in good order. When the body is in good order, then the *qi* is evenly distributed, which leads to unobstructed flow [of *qi*], which leads to the connection to the cosmic spirit (shen神), and in that state, there is nothing one cannot see, nothing one cannot hear, and nothing that can't be done. Therefore worries and disease cannot enter [the body], and evil *qi* cannot attack.[11]

When one can store and contain *qi* (and blood) within the five organs, the body actually becomes more self-sufficient. Furthermore, this energetic fuel improves the functioning of the body, where one becomes one with the cosmos, acquires limitless senses, and is protected from worries and diseases. In other words, a human body that is cultivated to have the ability to maintain adequate *qi* becomes not only connected to the cosmos but also shielded from illnesses. However, this state of enclosed self-sufficiency is technically hard to maintain:

When the essence (jing)[12] leaks at the eyes, then one sees clearly. When it is at the ears, one hears clearly. When it stays by the mouth, one speaks appropriate words. When it accumulates at the heart, one can see through worries. Therefore to close these four gateways will result in no troubles in the body. The hundred joints will not catch illness. It is neither death, nor life; not depleted [of *qi*] nor filled with it. This is the True Man.[13]

For one to conceive the world through bodily senses, it is necessary to bring the *qi* to reach outward, or for *qi* to "leak" from the body. The closed system will become free of troubles and illness, but "it is neither death, nor life." The True Man is therefore beyond living and dying, but has no interaction with anything outside of his body at all.

Therefore, to be a human who lives in the world, one's body is essentially a leaky container that needs to be refilled constantly. The Inner Classic has a more moderate model of keeping the task possible:

With all that shares the heavenly *qi*, keep clear and calm to manage one's thoughts, keep unobstructed to strengthen the *yangqi*, then even thieves and evil cannot cause harm.[14]

This involves both mental cultivation, "managing one's thoughts," and physical cultivation, "strengthening the *yangqi*." Both are considered to be cultivating the *qi* within the body. The mental cultivation tames the *qi* from being turbulent and leaking faster than it should.

Recall again that the *jing-qi-shen* trio is one essence in different manifestations across the spectrum of level of refinement, with *jing* as the most crude and material state, and *shen* as the most refined and thus immaterial state. The individual refinement of *qi* requires cultivation on all levels, and potentially also involves lifestyle changes:

In the management of the body, the best approach is to nourish the spirit (shen), and second to that is to nourish the physical form

> (xing).... When the spirit is clarified, one's ambition is tamed, all the joints [in the body] are at peace. This is the basis of nourishing one's character. To fatten up the flesh, fill up the abdomen, and to give in to desires and addictions, that's the worst way of nourishing life. [15]

Notice how ambition, which is a mental attribute, is associated with the state of the joints in the physical body. Also, filling the body with crude food rather than refined *qi* is "the worst way of nourishing life." The Inner Classic also suggests that the proper mental attitude can protect one from physical disease:

> Simplicity, contentment, and lack of desires... [these are qualities] that attract the true cosmic *qi*. When one guards the spirit inside, where can disease possibly come from? [16]

And of course, cultivation of *qi* at any level contributes to less turbulence in the shared *qi* in the shared space, with other people.

Health of the Shared Qi

In the TCM clinics in the Bay Area, practitioners not only train their patients to sense *qi* for validation of their healing, sometimes they also teach patients how to cultivate themselves to tap into the *qi* sources. Ashley, who leads *qigong* practices weekly, articulates how the refilling is done:

> When you do these simple movements, you gather the *qi* around you, from nature. There is a lot of *qi* out there, and you feel it, touch it, and you can even gather it up like a ball. You take some in, and you give some back too. And this is why it is also good to practice as a group—you cultivate together and everybody's *qi* becomes stronger.

It is understood that not only is this natural resource accessible for all with some training, collective cultivation of *qi* also helps amplify and purify the communal energy. Practitioners heal and educate the patients, and the patients can also participate in the greater project of healing and protecting the environment, not just conceptually and behaviorally, but also energetically. The mere act of practicing *qigong* in a group is contributing to the greater good by strengthening, and hopefully purifying, the communal *qi*.

I practiced *qigong* with Ashley and her group of friends and patients every weekend for about a year. Ashley tried to gather the group in a local park when the weather permitted, typically between April and November. The park was blessed with some areas ideal for group practice. There was an area that has a field circled by about twenty-five ginkgo trees that change leaf colors in the fall and bear an incredible amount of ginkgo fruits. Ginkgo leaves are known for their medicinal quality in many parts of Asia, and the nuts are considered a delicacy in Asian cuisines. Standing among these majestic, bountiful trees, the community of *qigong* practice included both the humans and the trees. Ashley encouraged a reciprocal, communal approach to *qi* cultivation, which was to not only gather *qi* from nature, but also share the refined *qi* with others. When the slightly chilly breeze of early autumn rattled the tree leaves, that same breeze brushed against our skins. When squirrels jumped from tree branch to tree branch, and quarreled in their small squeaky voices, somehow I heard them more clearly than I usually could. Another field that we frequented in the park had amaryllis, a half-translucent pink flower that would bloom on a single pink stem from the ground with no green leaves, blossoming in the fall as well. For about three weeks that we practiced in that field, these oddly fanciful blooms accompanied us with their quiet yet gently vibrant presence. In our thirty minutes of the freestyle meditation segment, we stood and focused on sensing the flow of *qi* in and around us. I can still remember fleeting moments of feeling extremely close to the flowers, as if I could touch the very essence of life in them.

At the end of these *qigong* practice sessions, sometimes group members would stay and briefly talk about their experiences. Most said they felt relaxed and energized after the session. Some members of the group actually felt the flow of *qi* around them, while others merely enjoyed being quiet and calm. One woman also noticed heightened sensory alertness; several times she complained that the road traffic (the locations we practiced in were quite far from the street side of the park), passing children, and dog barks in the neighborhood were especially loud and distracting when she was in the meditative state.

I asked Ashley how she felt when she went into the meditative state. She said she usually tried to casually feel the flow around her, but shared one incident that she thought was especially interesting. Ashley practices *qigong* at home daily, sometimes in her backyard but often inside her house. One day she practiced in her living room, and heard her husband coming home from work while she was in the meditative trance. She continued to practice as usual, with her eyes closed, but wondered why her husband seemed to walk straight by her without stopping. After she was done with the exercise, she found her husband in the kitchen, who was surprised that she was home. Apparently, her husband had walked into the living room and passed by her because he did not see her there at all. "What do you think happened?" I asked. "I'm not sure," Ashley pondered, "but maybe for a few moments in that *wuji* 無極 [non-polarized] state, I disappeared?" This is actually similar to the philosophical Daoist description of synchronization with the cosmos that I quoted in the previous chapter, where one's different senses all merge together, and the physical form dissipates into thin air.[17]

Although not all *qigong* practitioners share Ashley's experience, the understanding is that cultivation of individual *qi*, not only physically but mentally, is beneficial not only for the self but also for all that share the same universal *qi*. Besides maintaining daily *qigong* exercise, Ashley also practices *pigu* 辟穀 (abstaining from grains) once a year. Ashley is already a vegetarian and eats very light and healthy. But during her *bigu*, she eats minimal food and no grains at all for forty-nine consecutive days. This diet is an advanced part of her training with a *qigong* master from China. Recall that *jing* is the essence of digested food, and grains (*gu* 穀) are one of the main sources of *jing* in the human body. Daoist inner alchemists would try to advance their own bodies by using *qi* as the main source of functional energy instead of using *jing* as the main fuel. The physiological transformation would be significant for Ashley especially because she uses medical *qigong* extensively in her clinical practice. The more purified her *qi* is, the more effective the healing would be after she infuses *qi* into her patients. And the more she is able to constantly replenish *qi* into her own body, the more she has to offer in her healing.

One basic way that a TCM practitioner attempts to make energetic improvement on the communal level is to affect the *qi* of his patients, one by one. Most of the TCM practitioners I surveyed and interviewed do try to improve their own *qi* and physical strength, not just for their own protection from diseased *qi*, but also to increase therapeutic efficacy of their treatments on the patients. Leon Hammer considers that approach the defining quality of TCM as a healing art:

> There is a basic conflict between technology and art in the healing process. Technology insists that, as a test of the validity of the healing modality, the healer must not be essential to the healing process. However, in a healing system in which the movement and balance of energy is the critical factor in sickness and health, the energy of the healer always enters significantly into the system as a positive or negative force. In such a system, the healer is a significant factor in the healing process. His intention and his life-force influence the energy of the patient.[18]

Also, as we have seen in previous chapters, the practitioners, although in varying degrees, try to provide a transformative environment in the clinic. It would be fair to say that since TCM practitioners approach healing from the health side of the spectrum, the healing processes benefit from a healthful clinic environment and the healers' own well-balanced, abundantly filled, and appropriately grounded presence.

HEALTH AS EMPOWERMENT WITH SELF-KNOWLEDGE

The other half of the "teamwork" in the TCM clinic is the recognition of the role of the patient in providing her subjective perspective in the healing process. When the patient is taught to pay attention to her bodily sensations and to articulate those attentions through the rhetoric of *qi* and balance, the healer and the patient enter a discourse of interpreting and analyzing the patient's self-knowledge of the body. The patient's perception of her own well-being serves as an important basis for both diagnosis and healing, and therefore the self-knowledge of the patient is often at the core of the treatments.

A typical session in a TCM clinic takes from one to two hours. After the greetings, the practitioner tries to diagnose the patient's condition of the day. Patients who are in the middle of an ongoing set of treatments or who visit regularly for a "tune up" debrief on their self-observations since the last visit. When the healer starts the actual treatment, depending on the modalities used and the personalities of the healer and patient, types of conversations vary. Some healers choose to leave the room after acupuncture needles are inserted, and only return to check after fifteen to thirty minutes. During that time, the patient is left alone in the treatment room unless otherwise requested; according to some practitioners, during the process of unblocking the meridians, diseased *qi* is also released and dispersed from the patient's body. Staying in the room only increases the practitioner's exposure to diseased *qi*. Other healers who incorporate counseling and spiritual guidance techniques in their treatments, however, would stay in the room for conversations during the wait time for acupuncture.

Aside from allowing the TCM practitioners to schedule patients at thirty-minute intervals while still doing hour-long sessions, there are therapeutic benefits for the practice. Part of managing the *qi* is to keep it calm so as not to disperse it outward more than necessary. Some practitioners argue that talking during the treatment often results in aroused emotions in the patient, which is not an ideal state for the healing session. Even the herbalists who do not practice manual modalities ask the patients to sit quietly for a few minutes before they start the pulse diagnosis, so that the patient's *qi* is not so turbulent as to affect the pulse reading. Furthermore, being in the treatment room alone allows the patient time and space to observe and reflect on her own body. Some are finally able to relax and sleep for a short period of time. Some try to sense and observe their own physical sensations so that they can report back to the healer.

Because the sensations of the patient are taken as an important measurement for the efficacy of the treatment, the patient is empowered to voice his opinion on his own body, and encouraged to participate in the process of health maintenance. After all, nobody and nothing else can replace the patient's subjective perspective of well-being, and that transfers both the responsibility and control back to the patient from the healer and the system. Whereas the biomedical standard for judging whether one is ill is by looking at how deviated one is from the average within a population, TCM's standard is by the state of balance within each individual. That state of balance is much harder to achieve and maintain than is the lack of negative symptoms or stability in the body system. The equilibrium between the five elements and the *yin* and *yang* is essentially a moving target, where the human body is always subject to the influences of the all things external (what goes on in the surroundings, what food gets eaten, and so on) and all things internal (natural dispositions, preferences, histories, and memories). The TCM practitioner is able to observe from external signs and symptoms. However, since health is nothing short of complete balance, the patient needs to be able to articulate where he is feeling "off" so that he and the healer can work together to shift the body as closely toward the state of equilibrium as possible.

THE SEARCH FOR ULTIMATE HEALTH

In their services to the culturally, socially, and economically diverse patient base, TCM practitioners venture between cultures and medical systems to help themselves and their patients understand, interpret, and define "health."

However, real health in TCM is an impossible goal to attain: the ultimate healthy body is self-sufficient—effectively interconnected with the cosmic *qi*, with *qi* flowing effortlessly and without blockage inside the body and forming a protective layer outside the body. Furthermore, the body must be balanced between *yin* and *yang* and between the elements. By correspondence, different manifestations of *qi* and different dimensions of human experience must also be balanced. The human body is classically viewed as a leaky container that must be constantly refilled; the container is multilayered and needs to be constantly adjusted.

Furthermore, as we have discussed in the previous chapter, the quality of *qi* is also subject to constant refinement. The more refined the *qi* is, the less physical and more efficient it will become. When *qi* is at its most refined state, it becomes spirit. A human who successfully transforms all his *qi* into spirit can transcend the physical body and the differentiations between boundaries and dimensions. The Daoist inner alchemists used physical exercises, meditations, and herbs to help themselves in the process of such refinement; many of the methods that they used became the basis of TCM modalities. Although few patients walk into a TCM clinic with the goal of becoming immortals who are one with the cosmos, many do visit their TCM practitioners regularly for health maintenance and disease prevention. Some even learn cultivation techniques from their TCM practitioners and other local cultivation masters. With continuous balancing and refinement of *qi*, the practitioners and patients are inevitably on the spiritual (as in containing more refined, *shen*-type *qi* rather than *jing*-type *qi*) path of longevity, a prerequisite for immortality.

NOTES

1. See WHO webpage for its definition of health: http://www.who.int/about/definition/en/print.html.
2. See NIH website: http://health.nih.gov/.
3. Leon Hammer, *Dragon Rises and Red Bird Flies: Psychology and Chinese Medicine* (Barrytown, NY: Station Hill Press, 1990), 39–40.
4. Hammer, 39.
5. Hammer, 54.
6. *Huangting Neijing Jing*, chapter 7, "Zhidao 至道": 髮神蒼華字太元，腦神精根字泥丸，眼神明上字英玄，鼻神玉壟字靈堅，耳神空閑字幽田，舌神通命字正倫，齒神崿鋒字羅千。一面之神宗泥丸，泥丸九真皆有房，方圓一寸處此中，同服紫衣飛羅裳。但思一部壽無窮，非各別住俱腦中，列位次坐向外方，所存在心自相當。
7. Huangdi Neijing Lingshu, chapter 12, "Jingshui 經水."
8. Personal interview, October 18, 2008.
9. Paul Unschuld, "Chinese Medicine and Western Healthcare systems: Is Integration Possible?" (Public lecture in Berkeley, CA, November 11, 2008).
10. Personal communication, September 23, 2008.
11. Huainanzi, chapter 7, "Jingshen Xun 精神訓": 夫血氣能專於五藏而不外越，則胸腹充而嗜欲省矣。胸腹充而嗜欲省，則耳目清，聽視達矣。耳目清，聽視達，謂之明。…精神盛而氣不散則理，理則均，均則通，通則神，神則以視無不見， 以聽無不聞也，以為無不成也。是故憂患不能入也，而邪氣不能襲。
12. Again, it is important to remember that the *jing-qi-shen* trio are differentiated but at times also used interchangeably in classical discussions; in this passage, *jing* indicates that it is *qi* that is more on the material end of the scale.
13. Huainanzi, chapter 8, "Benjing Xun本經訓": 精泄於目，則其視明；在於耳，則其聽聰；留於口，則其言當；集於心，則其慮通。故閉四關則身無患，百節莫苑，莫死莫生，莫虛莫盈，是謂真人。
14. *Huangdi Neijing Suwen*, chapter 3, "Shengqi Tongtian生氣通天": 蒼天之氣，清靜則志意治，順之則陽氣固，雖有賊邪，弗能害也。
15. Huainanzi, chapter 20, "Taizu Xun泰族訓": 治身，太上養神，其次養形.... 神清志平，百節皆寧，養性之本也；肥肌膚，充腸腹，供嗜欲，養生之末也。
16. *Huangdi Neijing Suwen*, chapter 1, "Shanggu Tianzhen上古天真": 恬淡虛無，真氣從之，精神內守，病安從來。
17. In *Liezi*, as cited in the previous chapter: "Thereafter the eyes are like the ears, the ears are like the nose, and nose are like mouth; they are not differentiated. The heart-mind is consolidated, but the form dissipates, and the bones and flesh completely dissolve away."
18. Hammer, 9.

THIRTEEN
Concluding Analysis

Chinese ethnic practitioners, especially those who were trained in Mainland China, consider themselves the authentic knowledge brokers of TCM. Authenticity—here grounded in Chinese fluency, Chinese cultural competency, and PRC-TCM training—provides authority in TCM. This authority by authenticity is highly respected by non-Chinese ethnic practitioners as well. Those who have trained or interned in Mainland China, have Chinese ethnic mentors, or have the language skills to speak and read Chinese are considered more credible professionally. Authenticity is not the only source of power. If it were, there would be no innovation in TCM practices in the Bay Area.

The state licensing of acupuncture in California provides a basis for professional authority among TCM practitioners across ethnicities. Other resources and methods are actively and often creatively drawn from and utilized to strengthen clinical efficacy (as perceived and experienced by practitioners and patients) and to foster trusting relationships between practitioners and patients. Individual practitioners may or may not directly address the spiritual dimension in their clinical practices. However, in the collective discourse within the TCM profession, the non-parallel understandings of the "spiritual" dimension of the medicine between the Chinese and mainstream American cultural adherents create a categorical grey area where contesting interpretations and power negotiations take place. If the speeches and behaviors of TCM practitioners can be observed and framed as performances on the stage of the clinics, I press forward to argue that, in the production of such clinical performances, several identifiable patterns have developed as the healing practices successfully transfer across cultural boundaries to reach their desired audience.

(RE)CONNECTING IDEOLOGIES AND BELIEFS TO TCM PRACTICES

Rather than recognizing the whole traditional Chinese medical system, which includes different and often clashing views of the human body, health, and illness from mainline biomedicine, the state of California recognizes only acupuncture, and only as a modality. Before the year 2000, when California started to require clinical training for biomedical doctors to practice acupuncture, any biomedical doctor could use acupuncture as a modality clinically without prior training. The implication here is that acupuncture as a modality can be stripped of the worldview from which it emerged; yet its effectiveness, even outside of its original context, proves its true efficacy. This implication is supported by the fact that the National Institute of Health offers grants for research on the effectiveness of acupuncture, but only when it is done within the framework of Western science, and with the endorsement of biomedicine.

Although TCM schools in the Bay Area provide training where the treatment modalities are informed by the TCM theories, the larger societal location of TCM within the American medical hierarchy concurrently defines acupuncture as not necessarily attached to, or sometimes intentionally detached from, TCM theories; this is especially prominent in acupuncture practiced within major biomedical institutions. The conceptual separation between treatment modality and medical ideology prompts some practitioners to want to not only re-establish the connection between TCM practices and TCM theories, but also to create space for making new connections between practices and ideologies that were not previously related.

The attempts to "reconnect" can be seen in the acupuncturists' methods of personal cultivation; the term "cultivation" here is defined by a general common understanding of personal practices that elevate energy or promote personal health. In my 2006 California survey, 90 percent of my respondents said that they have some sort of personal cultivation, ranging from simply getting in touch with nature, to *qigong* and other specifically *qi*-oriented cultivations, to physical exercise that makes them more in tune with their own bodies. About 90 percent of those who responded to that particular survey item believed that, by increasing their own energy level, and for some even having more effective and direct use of their energy, their acupuncture needling in turn becomes more effective. The data indicate that 1) there is a common belief among practitioners that there is a connection between personal cultivation to increase their own energy levels and the effectiveness of their clinical practices; and 2) within the common belief of such a connection between personal cultivations and clinical practices, there is a wide range of interpretations as to exactly what the connection is and how the connection can be established.

While reconnections manifest in the plethora of approaches TCM practitioners use to increase their clinical efficacies, there seems to be a concurrent movement to simplify the theoretical interpretations of TCM practices. Specifically, the general energy paradigm of American alternative medicines is used as the lens through which the much more nuanced Chinese culturally based *qi* paradigm is understood. Both Chinese ethnic and non-Chinese ethnic practitioners try to understand new systems by comparing, contrasting, and analogizing with what they already know. In Ted Kaptchuk's *The Web That Has No Weaver*, an overview of TCM theories and practices so popular that it was often the first title that rolled off my informants' tongues, he starts with contrasting TCM against Western medicine.[1] In an older classic in American TCM, *Celestial Lancets* by Lu Gwei-djen and Joseph Needham, the authors not only explain TCM theories through biomedical vocabulary and frameworks, they also attempt to Latinize their English translations of the meridians, organs, and other physiological terms.[2]

Among my informants, I have seen practitioners who were previously trained in biomedicine and Western sciences interpreting TCM through those particular lenses. There are also practitioners who are non-Chinese and have their previous training in fields outside of biomedicine and Western sciences, and they tend to incorporate a mixture of vocabulary from common biomedical terminologies, energy paradigm, and popular spirituality, especially when they attempt to explain TCM concepts to their patients. For those Chinese ethnic practitioners who were previously trained in other professional disciplines, this is also the case when they approach biomedicine. Chinese ethnic practitioners, especially those trained in China, also use their existing knowledge to approach other alternative medical systems. Depending on their medical trainings (if they were trained predominantly in biomedicine, or in TCM, or an integration of both), I have heard practitioners use a combination of biomedical and TCM frameworks and concepts known in the Chinese culture to talk about homeopathy and crystal healing. As a result of constant and ongoing cross-cultural comparisons between similar yet different concepts such as *qi*, energy, magnetic fields, pneuma, and so on, the emphases on similarities or overlaps between theoretical systems are often hastily taken as equating categories across systems. In other words, analogies that were first meant to help understandings across boundaries are being taken as equivalents, where differences and nuances are glossed over or ignored completely. For instance, most TCM practitioners in the Bay Area, regardless of ethnicities, would readily agree to the statement that "*qi* is like energy" without giving much more thought about how the two categories differ in many ways. I argue that there is now, at least at the ground level of everyday interactions in the TCM clinics, a more globalized, syncretic, and generally more simplistic understanding of each of these separate systems that is popularly understood in terms of energy.

From this basic and agreed-upon understanding of *qi* that is accessible to most practitioners and patients even without Chinese cultural and linguistic competency, the TCM community as a whole then continues to engage with *qi* in deeper ways, whether through validation by biomedical clinical trials, explorations into Chinese medical classics, or verifications by somatic experiences.

Experiential Dimension of TCM Healing Brings About Ideological Conversion

We have seen in the previous chapters that, being practitioners of an alternative medicine in the United States, the TCM practitioners have various approaches to enhance their professional images, business success, and clinical efficacy. While "spiritual" may or may not be the center of attention of all TCM practitioners I talked to, an important characteristic that is shared by all is the importance of the experiential dimension, not only in their clinical practices, but also in their own entry points into the medicine and interpretations of healing.

The emphasis on the experiential dimension of clinical treatment is expressed through the attention to the clinic environment and treatment procedures to ensure not only that the treatment is physically therapeutic, but also that the experience of the treatment is comfortable, calming, and emotionally positive. Beyond merely the perceived expectations of the consumerist market (consisting of the demands of the patients and limitations placed by health insurance providers), the life stories of the practitioners reveal a strong relationship between their own experiential encounters with TCM treatments and their entries into the profession. This relationship is especially prevalent among non-Chinese practitioners, who often recount their personal experiences with TCM treatments as patients themselves as the turning points of their professional lives. The efficacy of the treatments they received became the first highly subjective validation of the efficacy of TCM. Without actually labeling it "religious conversion," perhaps the experientially based validation can be likened to the process of religious conversion,[3] which, without the "religious" part of it, can be seen as a process of ideological conversion. It is a conversion not only from biomedicine to TCM, but also from a lack of awareness toward one's body and the surrounding environment to a conscious and responsible way of living and being. This is related to the reconnection between ideology and practice, where in this instance, a whole holistic lifestyle ideology is attached to TCM practices to create a clinical package.

As these "personally converted" practitioners introduce TCM treatments to their non-Chinese patients, they also foster this "conversion" process by encouraging experiential validation of clinical efficacy. As discussed previously, practitioners actively train patients to recognize and articulate TCM categories of subtle sensations, most notably but not limited to sensations related to *qi* movements. The sensation of *deqi* and physically observable signs of it (red, swelling, and increased temperature on the skin around the insertion point), which happen as a needle is properly inserted into an acupuncture point, are used as obvious and clearly scientific evidence that the needles are working properly. The patients are also encouraged to pay attention to their own physical sensations during treatment sessions and between treatments. While the practitioners may very well be asking for the patients' perspectives only as a basis of diagnosis and for design of treatments, the validation of the patients' subjective sensations empowers the patients in the clinical encounters.

When the practitioners allow space for extensive conversations, the attention on physical sensations seems to easily lead patients to revelations on emotional, psychological, and other non-physical issues. Some practitioners include counseling as part of their scope of practice, but perhaps many of the patients already have a preconceived expectation that TCM as a holistic medicine does not exclude beyond-physical issues. Indeed, practitioners who are open to such conversations (such as Crystal, in chapter 2, and Thomas, in chapter 5) often find themselves healing psychological traumas that were first disguised as physical symptoms.[4] Whereas biomedical physicians would probably refer these patients to psychotherapists or psychiatric specialists, the TCM practitioners do not typically refer their patients out of their practices.[5] As a result, veteran TCM practitioners have their loyal customers often because they not only heal physical conditions, but they are there for the patients' emotional, psychological, and even spiritual struggles.

SPIRITUAL ASPECT OF TCM CLINICAL CONTEXT

In the attempt to create the space for my informants to come forward with their own conceptions and voices, I started my fieldwork with an intentionally open definition for "spirituality." The merely suggestive framing of "spirituality" was articulated as: "the seeking of the experience in the connection with what is larger/more than oneself—with nature, with the supernatural, with a community of people, or with another individual, and/or also seeking the experience of transformation as a result of that connection."

Those practitioners who locate themselves within or close to the biomedical institutions and/or the "scientific" theoretical orientation are less inclined to emphasize their personal spiritual beliefs or to incorporate energetic or other non-physical healing modalities into their clinical practices. Those practitioners who locate themselves as alternatives to the biomedical and mainstream American norm are more inclined to incorporate spiritual approaches. The majority of my informants locate between the extremes: most practitioners are not completely against the idea of incorporating spiritual healing when circumstances demand, but neither do they rely exclusively on spiritual methods for clinical treatments or business success.

While the institutional training of TCM clearly neither includes nor encourages religious or spiritual methods in TCM clinical practices, individual practitioners may choose to incorporate their religious, spiritual, or psychic beliefs and practices into their clinical practices. There is a wide range of how these beliefs and practices are included clinically. As mentioned in the previous section, TCM practitioners in the Bay Area connect and reconnect ideologies and theories to their clinical practices. Some practitioners see these religious, spiritual, and psychic beliefs, abilities, and methods as part of their personal cultivations (see chapter 1 for survey results). In instances where practitioners believe that personal cultivations are aimed to enhance their own personal well-being and indirectly improve their clinical efficacy, the patients are usually not explicitly informed of these "behind the scene" practices. Jason, who told me that he prays in a separate room when he encounters difficult cases, prays to gain more strength to treat his patients to the best of his abilities. The prayers are not part of the treatments, and he does not always disclose his praying practice to the patients he prays for.

Among the practitioners who say that they chant Buddhist mantras during treatments, Ashley is the only one who would chant out loud and encourage her patients to chant with her—but only when she is sure that they are receptive and willing. Most other practitioners say they chant to themselves, silently and undisclosed to their patients. My interpretation of this latter approach is that the practitioners chant in the hope of maximizing the efficacy of their treatments, but do not wish to be mistaken by their patients as lacking medical competency and relying only on wishful thinking. Most importantly, practitioners are aware of the mainstream American stigma toward spiritual healing (for example, Joy's story in chapter 6, in which her patients' pastor warned her of suspicious healing methods). Those practitioners who have psychic abilities typically do not disclose those abilities to their patients, mostly due to their concern of a stigma on psychic healers.

While practitioners express that the patients may not appreciate knowing that non-medical healing is involved in their treatments, some practitioners, especially non-Chinese practitioners, decorate their clinics with religious symbols (Tibetan *tangkas*, small Buddhist statues, and Daoist paintings are popular), and analyze the non-physical dimensions of their patients' conditions with insights that seem to come from their own spiritual ponderings (attachment for the Buddhists, and pollutions and contaminations for the eco-activists). In other words, while directly applying non-medical techniques clinically is commonly uncalled for, it is perfectly acceptable, if not preferred, that a practitioner herself appears wise or enlightened. Perhaps part of that "wise and enlightened" through religious and cultural symbols (usually Tibetan Buddhist or Daoist) taps directly into the Orientalist fantasies of both the patients and the practitioners.

The TCM practitioners' attention to creating a certain clinic atmosphere, as demonstrated by my survey results, individual clinic visits, and the TCM school classes and clinics, is related to the experiential-spiritual aspect of the TCM clinical practices. On the one hand, one can argue that creating a comfortable, soothing, and relaxing environment for clinical treatments has nothing to do with the "spiritual." On the other hand, the intention to create transformative experiences for the patients (even just going from stressed to relaxed), sometimes leads to experiences for the patients and even practitioners that they later consider spiritual. For example, one practitioner told me a story of his patient describing the experience "like flying" during an acupuncture treatment. An example of a practitioner articulating a spiritual experience in the clinic is Rafael, who in chapter 6 shared that he felt that he was one with the patients when he treated them. Intriguingly, those who are more willing to explore and exercise the "spiritual" dimension of their clinical practices don't necessarily see themselves as in opposition to biomedicine; a more accurate description of their perceived relation to biomedicine may be that they offer more of themselves in healing compared to biomedical physicians. Beyond the regular clinical procedures, many TCM practitioners spend much time and effort in improving the quality of qi in their own body (through cultivation) and in the clinic (through attention to details) for additional therapeutic benefits. Some practitioners (such as Alison and Rafael, in chapter 8) also feel that they need to be focused and attuned to the patients to provide effective healing.

In the context of TCM theories and practices, since qi is the basic material for all things in the universe, it is also a freely accessible resource for all. TCM practitioners cultivate themselves to stay connected to the qi in nature and in other beings around them. They often also train their patients to sense, cultivate, refine, and use qi to improve their health. Qi, with the non-material/spiritual as one of its dimensions, is essentially a resource that can be tapped into. What is interesting about qi as resource is that, in the scope of the cosmos as a whole, it is limitless in quantity. Furthermore, it is a resource that can be accessed and used by anyone who has been trained. And because qi transcends forms and boundaries, it can be transformed from one dimension to another. The passage between dimensions also means that qi can be converted between forms and exchanged across boundaries.

In the previous chapters, I demonstrated that TCM practitioners, especially but not exclusively the Chinese ethnic practitioners among them, using qi sensations as evidence, understand qi as a matter that is an extension of the physical rather than nonphysical or beyond physical. On the other hand, *qi*, as the cosmically shared matter of all dimensions, fits into the spiritual category. *Huangdi Neijing Suwen* famously states that "by following the sequence of the seasons and the patterns of the *qi* of heaven, one can *"tong shenming* 通神明."[6] *Tong shenming* here can be variously interpreted as "connecting to and communicating with the deities (*shenming* 神明)," "clearing of the channels to achieve clarity in one's *shen*," and perhaps "attaining the state of luminousness which allows one access to the miraculous." Whether *shenming* or *shen* and *ming* should be understood as spiritual categories is debatable, because it depends on how one perceives the distinction between physical and non-physical. The shared and connective nature of *qi* makes such distinction hazy, if not altogether ambiguous. On the other hand, because the existence of *qi* can only be indirectly demonstrated through physiological changes and trained sensations, the invisible matter is often dismissed as a mere "belief" by those who lack the physical sensation of *qi* and have no control over it as a source of vitality and healing power.

Some practitioners from China readily recognize the importance of *qi* in their practices and in the TCM theories, but at the same time vehemently attack the usage of *qigong* as the main business attraction or treatment modality. Incidentally, those who are most vocal against *qigong* treatments are also state-trained from China who have worked and taught in medical schools there. The recent history of governmental control over *qigong* practices[7] and the prosecution of *Falungong* 法輪功 practitioners in Mainland China may have something to do with these Chinese immigrant practitioners' actively distancing themselves from *qigong* treatments. Within the American context, it may also be a strategy by these practitioners to further consolidate their authorities as "those who were truly properly trained," evidenced by their accusation that *qigong* healers are all charlatans.

Non-Chinese practitioners carry with them a different set of baggage: "spirituality" is a well-established category that comes with mixed blessings. The perceived social stigma toward religious, spiritual, and psychic healing is carefully observed and sometimes brilliantly manipulated by the TCM practitioners.

Besides the experiential-spiritual, many non-Chinese practitioners also expand the possibility of the healing by cultivating and demonstrating transcultural insights. While Chinese ethnic and especially China-trained practitioners assert their professional authority through cultural authenticity, some of the non-Chinese practitioners establish their authority by demonstrating to their patients and students that their cultivated insights effectively cut across cultural divides and see the universal nature of what is human. These insights may result from cultural immersion, language mastery, years of tireless individual study, and extensive clinical experiences, but often the hints of religious symbols reinforce if not enhances the image of insightfulness. Very often (but not always), such insight is closely linked to or even merges with the practitioners' psychic abilities.

Here I suggest that we broaden the category of "spiritual" to include the spectrum across the Chinese and mainstream American cultures, rather than using either cultural definition as standard against the other. Without drawing definitive boundaries as to where the "spiritual" may end, much of what is considered in the Western world emotional, psychological, and experiential—those human experiences that are subjective and beyond merely what is physical, visible, and measurable—can arguably be considered "spiritual" without necessarily having religious connotations. From the Chinese side, the cosmological correspondences across dimensions and categories of bodily sensations that are not only experientially based but also require certain cultural competency in traditional Chinese worldviews and cosmological concepts to articulate should also qualify as possibly "spiritual." Furthermore, as I have suggested in chapters 11 and 12, the process of refining the *qi* from its material state to the metaphysical manifestation is also inevitably spiritual. In essence, I argue for not only the recognition that "spiritual" is understood differently across the cultural divide, but also the sensitivity to include a wider range of possibilities of interpretations of spiritual categories.

With the above cross-cultural understanding of what is considered "spiritual," the spiritual resources and methods used in practices of TCM in the Bay Area can be roughly grouped into four categories: 1) sources that fall clearly into the religious categories, such as practices and rituals from institutionalized and recognized major religions; 2) psychic abilities and methods; 3) atmospheric elements in the clinical experience, such as clinic decor, lighting, music, and so on; and 4) *qi* and energy related sources that are seen as spiritual by some and cosmically physical by others.

While most resources are accessible and utilized by some and rarely by all, *qi* as a resource is theoretically accessible for all. With training in sensing and articulating the presence, movements, and qualities of *qi*, anyone can tap into the shared *qi* in our surroundings and in nature. This training is in itself a type of cultural competency, but a cultural competency that can be easily acquired provided that one has an open mind. By definition, there is no living person who has no *qi* already in her, and there is unlimited *qi* to connect to and gather in the cosmos. Conceptually, it is incredibly empowering for the practitioners and patients to connect to *qi* on the cosmic level, and to learn to cultivate the *qi* within themselves, in the human community and as part of nature. Medically, *qi* as the basic material for being is essential for the goal of ultimate health. The continual refinement of *qi* in different dimensions of human existence makes the physical body more efficient, and closer to the perfect balance that defines real health in TCM. Although ultimate health is next to impossible to achieve, *qi* is available for all to use as people work toward better health.

GLOBALIZATION, LOCALIZATION, OR GLOCALIZATION OF TCM

In this book, I presented how TCM crosses cultural boundaries in the San Francisco Bay Area, carefully contextualized in the local demographics, cultural dynamics, and history. It should be emphasized that the geographic framing does not mean that the practitioners are limited by the geography. In fact, most the TCM practitioners in my study are active participants in the global economy and exchanges. Chinese diasporan practitioners are not the only ones straddling between two cultures and travelling between the United States and Asia; many non-Chinese practitioners also seek opportunities to acquire medical, cultural, and linguistic knowledge that can bring them closer to the heart of the TCM theoretical system. At the very least, the herbs and patent formulae most practitioners prescribe to their patients are products of a vibrant international agricultural and pharmaceutical market.

In clinical interactions with patients and sometimes in educating the general public as well, TCM practitioners inevitably serve as representatives of the medicine and brokers of knowledge related to the medicine. TCM as a knowledge system and medical culture has been globalized. The mobility of today's world citizens deterritorialized[8] TCM from the limited geography of China and the limited ethnic-cultural context of Chinese subcultures into the United States and the American mainstream culture. At the same time, TCM is becoming localized as practitioners interpret TCM theories into practices that can best meet the healthcare needs of their patients. These two features together make what social scientists call glocalization: the simultaneous globalizing and localizing that sidesteps much of the control of the nation state.[9] While the state of California has control over licensing of the acupuncturists and the scope of their practice, localized political efforts have negotiated ample space for variety and creativity in the actual implementation of clinical TCM. Indeed, we have seen in this book the range of locations and styles among the practitioners that cater to the preferences and needs of numerous different market niches in the diverse Bay Area population.

Furthermore, the globalized knowledge production (although the production loop is still spotty) and localized sensitivities and reflections among TCM practitioners really become the grounds for the creolization of cultures. Of the different definitions of cultural creolization, Nicholas R. Spitzer has one that comes closest to the situation of the TCM practitioners in the Bay Area:

> Creolized societies conjoin two or more formerly discrete cultures in a new setting to create a social order in which heterogeneous

styles, structures, and contents are differentially preserved while becoming wholly constituted in and adapted to new circumstances with new and multifaceted meanings. Yet in all this, earlier cultural traditions, practices, symbols, and sensibilities are often maintained, revered, and even highlighted, though with transformed shades and subtleties of meaning.[10]

Perhaps the TCM practitioners are not culturally creolized in every aspect of their lives; there is no indication of emergent new hybrid ethnicity[11] out of this particular encounter between Chinese and American cultures. Nonetheless, within the limited role of being TCM practitioners, my informants are creolized in their cosmological beliefs, theoretical thinking, and clinical strategies.

Taking into consideration the complex power negotiations between different cultures, Ulf Hannerz further suggests that "the cultural processes of creolization are not simply a matter of constant pressure from the center toward the periphery, but a much more creative interplay."[12] Building on Hannerz's recognition of "creative interplay," now let us take one last look at the mechanism of power negotiation among the TCM practitioners within this ongoing process of creolization.

Edward Shils theorizes that a society is structured in terms of center and periphery, where the center is defined by a set of values considered as sacred. Each individual's power location within the society depends on the degree of commonality one has with the center; those more identical with the center are closer to the center, and those less identical with the center are further away.[13] When we look at the American society through Shils' model, we can actually see how assimilation is supposed to work. There is a set of American values and attributes that defines "American-ness," and those who are more identical to these core values and attributes, or more assimilated, are closer to the center compared to the unassimilated.

But that is too simplistic. The coexistence of two power centers in the Chinese diaspora is evident: as ethnic Chinese, one is subject to (but does not have to always abide by) the Chinese understanding of family obligations and filial duties, the expectation of familiarity with the Chinese language and etiquette, and the Chinese socio-familial network that both binds the community together and gives individual members access to all sorts of members-only benefits. As a resident[14] in American society, one is also expected to abide by the laws, understand English, and at least appreciate the social knowledge of being American.

The two power centers must complement each other out of necessity. Unless the host society deports the diasporans altogether, the Chinese diaspora exists within the American society in ways that the host society institutionally allows. In turn, the diaspora seeks to maximize its autonomy and distinctiveness within the space allowed by the host society. As an example, Amy Freedman finds that the Chinese diasporans participate in politics through mobilization efforts of community leaders when there are good incentives to do so, and form organizations depending on the problems that need to be overcome in order to achieve effective mobilization.[15] In a sense, the host society and the diaspora co-create the niches and boundaries of the diaspora.

As a community, the TCM practitioners all locate on two overlapping grids: one being the cultural grid affected by two cultural cores, and another being the ideological grid affected by the two medical systems and other healing-related ideologies that permeate the mainstream American culture. The practitioners collectively represent an institutionally standardized yet internally pluralistic medical system, and individually identify somewhere along this complex cultural-ideological matrix. The competitive consumerist market they work in demands that they not only uphold the institutional standard but also exceed the standard.

It is the interpretations, packaging, and presentations of their individual locations on the cultural-ideological matrix that set each successful[16] practitioner apart from the minimal standards of general training. This is where the effective incorporation of a wide range of healing methods becomes crucial in the survival of a TCM practitioner in the profession. Especially in the practitioners' use of spiritual healing, we have seen how flexible the practitioners are in going to all the possible resources that they have access to, and how creative they are in combining elements of different ideological systems into concrete practice.

At the same time, their practices are limited by the consumerist market, state regulations, and health insurance coverage. The responses of the patients are crucial in how much a practitioner utilizes spiritual methods. With patients who are receptive and interested, TCM practitioners use and even experiment with spiritual-related methods; otherwise the practitioners stay with only the standard modalities. The legal definitions and regulations by the state of California (and in turn the health insurance providers who interpret state regulations) regarding licensed acupuncturists set definite perimeters around not only the scope of practice but also acceptable treatment modalities.

It will be interesting to continue to observe the development of TCM in the Bay Area as part of the global TCM economy. How will the "on the ground" experiences, knowledge, and ideology developed in the Bay Area affect the outlook of TCM in China? How will TCM, now one of the most popular alternative and/or complementary medical systems in the United States, fare in the current national healthcare reform? If there is a "standard TCM" that has previously been defined by PRC-TCM, will the openness toward a spiritual (or at least beyond-physical) dimension by the TCM practitioners in the Bay Area induce significant global movements in the medical system away from obsessions with scientism and modernity?

What is clear is TCM, along with the Chinese diaspora, is here to stay as part of the American sociocultural landscape. It has been localized and homegrown, customized to the needs of Americans in all walks of life. TCM has become, as one practitioner says, "*qi*-fully yours."

NOTES

1. Ted J. Kaptchuk, *The Web That Has No Weaver: Understanding Chinese Medicine* (New York: McGraw-Hill, 2000).

2. Gwei-djen Lu and Joseph Needham, *Celestial Lancets: A History and Rationale of Acupuncture and Moxa* (Cambridge: Cambridge University Press, 1980).

3. Here I define "conversion" simply as a shift of identity from one tradition to another tradition. This is derived from the definition of religious conversion by Rodney Stark and Roger Finke, where they specify the shift to be across religious traditions. See Rodney Stark and Roger Finke, *Acts of Faith: Explaining the Human Side of Religion* (Berkeley: University of California Press, 2000), 114.

4. Also see Linda L. Barnes, "The Psychologizing of Chinese Healing Practices in the United States," *Culture, Medicine, and Psychiatry* 22 (1998): 412–43.

5. While practitioners sometimes refer patients to other TCM practitioners who have specializations, the current disconnect and power differential between TCM and the biomedical establishments gives TCM practitioners little authority, resource, or connections to make referrals to biomedical specialists directly.

6. *Huangdi Neijing Suwen*, chapter 2, "Siqi Tiaoshen 四氣調神." Following the proper sequence of the seasons and abiding to the qi of the heavens will lead to communication/clarification of *shenming* (因時之序，服天氣而通神明).

7. See Nancy N. Chen, *Breathing Spaces: Qigong, Psychiatry, and Healing in China* (New York: Columbia University Press, 2003).

8. See John Tomlinson, *Globalization and Culture* (Cambridge: Polity, 1999), 29–30; Jose Casanova, "Religion, the New Millennium, and Globalization," *Sociology of Religion* 62, no. 4 (2001): 429; Stanley J. Tambiah, "Transnational Movements, Diaspora, and Multiple Modernities," *Daedalus* 129, no. 1 (2000): 178.

9. This is Jose Casanova's definition of the term. See Casanova, "Religion, the New Millennium, and Globalization." For other variations, see Roland Robertson, "Glocalization: Time-Space and Homogeneity-Heterogeneity," in *Global Modernities*, ed. Mike Featherstone, Scott Lash, and Roland Robertson (London: Sage Publications, 1995), 25–44; Victor Roudometof, "Transnationalism, Cosmopolitanism and Glocalization," *Current Sociology* 53, no. 1 (2005): 113–35; Richard Giulianotti and Roland Robertson, "Forms of Glocalization: Globalization and the Migration Strategies of Scottish Football Fans in North America," *Sociology of Religion* 41 (2007): 133–52.

10. Nicholas R. Spitzer, "Monde Créole: The Cultural World of French Louisiana Creoles and the Creolization of World Cultures," *Journal of American Folklore* 116, no. 459 (2003): 58–59.

11. See Frank Korom, "Memory, Innovation and Emergent Ethnicities," *Diaspora* 3, no. 2 (1994): 135–55.

12. Ulf Hannerz, *Cultural Complexity: Studies in the Social Organization of Meaning* (New York: Columbia University Press, 1992), 264–65.

13. See Edward Shils, *Center and Periphery: Essays in Macro Society* (Chicago: University of Chicago Press, 1975), 3–16.

14. By this I mean living here, whether legally or illegally.

15. Amy L. Freedman, *Political Participation and Ethnic Minorities: Chinese Overseas in Malaysia, Indonesia, and the United States* (New York: Routledge, 2000), 10–11, 19.

16. Success here is defined in a market-oriented sense, where a practitioner is able to stay competitive in the healthcare profession and sustain a livelihood by practicing TCM, regardless of the style or healing efficacy of their clinical practices.

Appendix

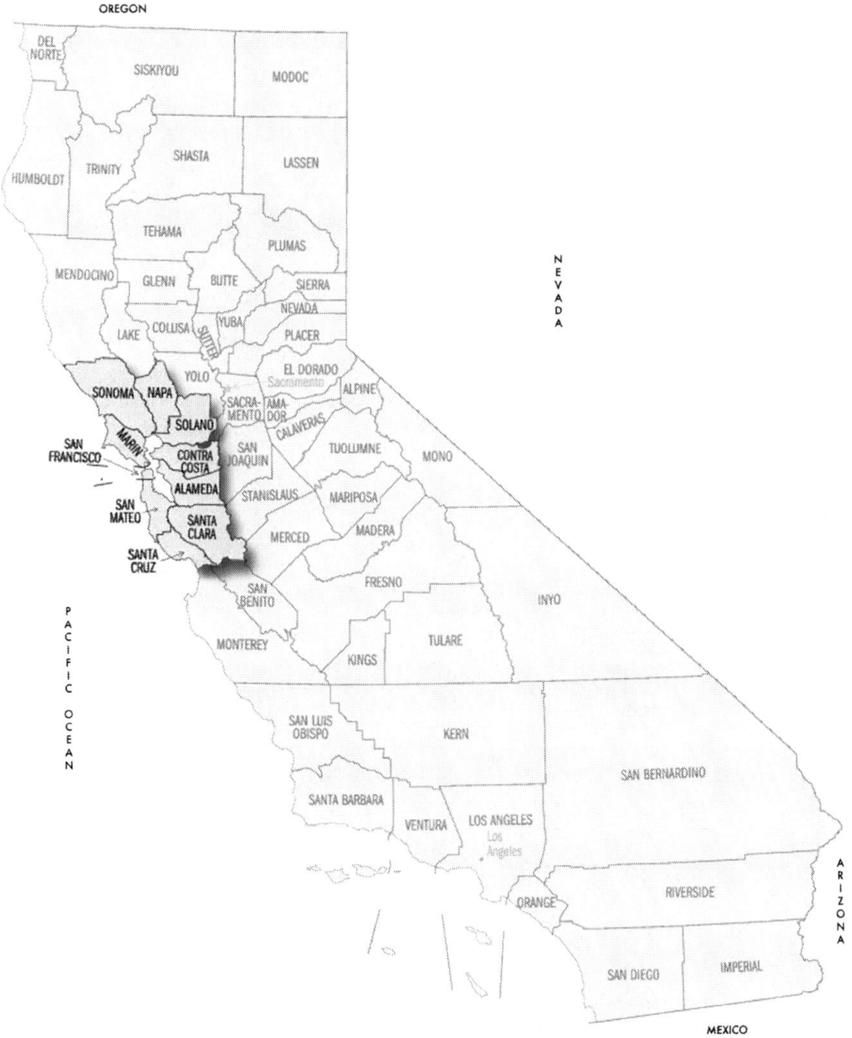

Figure 13.1. Map of San Francisco Bay Area Counties. The base map of all counties in California came from www.censusfinder.com/mapca.htm (accessed November 17, 2009), upon which I performed some digital alteration to showcase the counties covered in this study.

Table 13.1. Asian Pacific-Islander and White Populations in the Bay Area

	1990		2000		2008 (estimate)	
	10 counties	Core Bay	10 Counties	Core Bay	10 Counties	Core Bay
White	61%	54%	72%	66%	52%	52%
Asian Pacific Islander	15%	19%	20%	26%	36%	32%
Other	24%	27%	8%	8%	12%	16%

Core Bay includes the metropolitan areas of Oakland, San Francisco, and San Jose.

Table 13.2. Ethnicity

	Count	Percentage
Caucasian/European descent	56	41%
Chinese descent	60	44%
Korean descent	8	6%
Other Asian descent	6	4%
Latin descent	1	1%
African descent	2	1%
Native American descent	0	0%
Mixed ethnicities	5	4%
Total	138	100%

Table 13.3. Gender

	Count	Percentage
Male	55	40%
Female	72	52%
No response	11	8%
Total	138	100%

Table 13.4. Age

	Count	Percentage
34 and younger	7	5%
35-42	23	17%
43-61 ("Baby Boomers")	74	54%
62 and older	14	10%
No response	20	15%
Total	138	100%

The age categories were created after the survey results were calculated. The categories were made around the "Baby Boomers" category.

Table 13.5. Highest Level of Education Outside of TCM Training

	Count	Percentage
Associate of Arts (AA)	8	6%
Bachelors (BS/BA)	46	33%
Masters (MS/MA)	35	25%
PhD	12	9%
MD	8	6%
PhD + MD	2	1%
Other	8	6%
No response	19	14%
Total	138	100%

Appendix

Table 13.6. Words/Phrases That Best Describe Sources of or Causes to Human Illnesses.

	Count	Percentage
Unhealthy lifestyle	118	88%
Disharmony between body and mind	106	79%
Pathogens	87	65%
Pollutants and chemicals	81	60%
Blockage	64	48%
Negligence	50	37%
Imbalance in the environment	47	35%
Excess/deficiency	44	33%
Wind	43	32%
Desire	33	25%
Stress	5	4%
Injury	2	1%
Other	15	11%

Numbers calculated based on a sample size of 134; 4 (3%) out of 138 respondents did not respond to this question. Each respondent was asked to select all categories that apply, and therefore the categories do not produce mutually exclusive numbers.

Table 13.7. Do you utilize colors (especially the colors of the five elements) in your clinical treatments? If yes, how?

	Count	Percentage
No response	54	39%
No	58	42%
Yes	26	20%
Yes with no specific details	4	15%
Yes—in diagnosis	8	30%
Yes—in treatments	6	22%
Yes—in prescriptions	1	4%
Yes—for *fengshui*	4	15%
Yes—other	4	15%
Total responses for Yes (1 respondent lists 2 answers)	27	100%

Table 13.8. Was there any religious affiliation or spiritual identification in your household during your upbringing? What was it? And do you have any religious affiliation or spiritual identification now? What is it?

	Religious Identity/ Affiliation During Upbringing		Religious Identity/ Affiliation Now	
No response or not applicable	31	22%	31	22%
None	30	22%	24	17%
Christian	49	36%	26	19%
God	2	14%	6	4%
Buddhism	10	7%	20	14%
Judaism/Jew	7	5%	6	4%
Spiritual, but not religious	0	0%	3	2%
Eclectic	0	0%	8	6%
Other	9	7%	14	10%
Total	138	100%	138	100%

Table 13.9. Do you regularly practice any of the following? (Check all that apply and specify what type of each you practice.)

	Count	Percentage
Get in touch with nature	66	53%
Sitting meditation	46	37%
Qigong exercises	38	31%
Taichi exercises	35	28%
Pray to God/Allah/Goddess	31	25%
Communicate to spiritual beings or forces	31	25%
Yoga	29	21%
Qi cultivation	23	19%
Visualization	21	15%
Chant sutras or sacred names	14	11%
Chinese martial arts	13	10%
Incense offering	8	6%
Other	18	15%

Numbers calculated based on a sample size of 124; 14 (10%) out of 138 respondents did not respond to this question. Each respondent was asked to select all categories that apply, and therefore the categories do not produce mutually exclusive numbers.

Table 13.10. How important are the above practices to your clinical practice?

	Count	Percentages		
Not Relevant	12	10%	10%	10%
Between NR and SH	1	<1%	~18%	~90%
Somewhat Helpful	22	18%		
Between SH and VH	1	<1%	~72%	
Very Helpful	48	39%		
Between VH and EI	6	5%		
Extremely Important	33	27%		

Numbers calculated based on a sample size of 123; 15 (11%) out of 138 respondents did not respond to this question. Each respondent was asked to select all categories that apply, and therefore the categories do not produce mutually exclusive numbers.

Table 13.11. Do you have specific strategies to calm your patients? What do you do?

	Count	Percentage
Play music and/or natural sounds	119	89%
Scents/aromatherapy	23	17%
Use calming voice and attitude	91	68%
Imagine and/or visualize calmness	28	21%
Pray or chant during treatment	3	2%
Physical treatment/ comfortable environment	11	8%
Teach patient breathing strategy	7	5%
Other	7	5%

Numbers calculated based on a sample size of 133; 5 (4%) out of 138 respondents did not respond to this question. Each respondent was asked to select all categories that apply, and therefore the categories do not produce mutually exclusive numbers.

Table 13.12. Do you visualize or try to feel the movements of positive and negative energy when you treat patients? If you do, how?

	Count	Percentage
No response	50	36%
No	28	20%
Yes	60	43%
Yes with no specific details	6	10%
Yes—through senses/physical contact	29	47%
Yes—intention/imagination/visualization	15	24%
Yes—*qi* or energy transfer	3	5%
Yes—other	9	15%
Total responses for Yes (2 respondents list 2 answers each)	62	100%

Table 13.13. SF Bay Area Acupuncture Licensee Count (as of May 22, 2009)

County	License Issued	Active	Clear*	Inactive**	Delinquent	CEU*** Inadequate
Alameda	626	547	515	79	27	5
Contra Costa	163	135	132	28	2	1
Marin	204	183	159	21	19	5
Napa	20	19	18	1	1	
San Francisco	679	529	486	150	38	5
San Mateo	184	157	147	27	8	2
Santa Clara	553	487	462	66	21	4
Santa Cruz	255	222	208	33	11	3
Solano	21	16	15	5	1	
Sonoma	150	136	129	14	6	1
Total	**2,855**	**2,431**	**2,271**	**424**	**134**	**26**

Total number of licenses issued in California: 13,110.
*Inactive: Cancelled, Revoked, Deceased, Surrendered
**Clear: All requirements met and License fees paid
***CEU = Continuing Education Units

Table 13.14. Do you have (or would like to have) any of the following objects prominently displayed in your clinic/office? Check all that apply.

	Count	Percentage
Credentials and licenses	123	93%
Meridians and acupuncture points	101	77%
Water fountain and/or fish tank	64	48%
Western anatomy	46	35%
Five elements	26	20%
Aromatherapy	26	20%
Pictures and letters from patients	25	19%
Natural crystal	24	18%
Pictures of famous doctors and masters	10	8%
Other	1	<1%

Numbers calculated based on a sample size of 132; 6 (4%) out of 138 respondents did not respond to this question. Each respondent was asked to select all categories that apply, and therefore the categories do not produce mutually exclusive numbers.

Table 13.15. What are three adjectives you would want new clients to think of when they first walk into your clinic/office?

	Count	Percentage
Sanctuary	60	58%
Professional	51	50%
Approachable	43	42%
Clean	40	39%
Peaceful	31	30%
Comfortable	22	21%
Reliable	18	17%
Positive visual impressions and ambience	15	15%
High energy	5	5%
Other	8	8%
No response	35	25% (of total 138)

Out of 138 respondents, 35 (25%) did not respond to this question. Each respondent was asked to list three adjectives they want the clinic environment to conjure when a patient first walks in. Some respondents list words that I later categorize into the same categories, so percentages will not have much statistical value for this item.

Appendix 227

School	Year Established	Year Accredited	Degree Programs	Other Programs	Affiliations	Languages of Instruction
AIMC (Acupuncture & Integrative Medicine College) Berkeley	1990 (Meiji) 2004 (AIMC)	2004	MSOM (Master of Science in Oriental Medicine)	Certificates: Asian Bodywork; Tuina; Medical Qigong; Japanese Acupuncture; Continued Education; Public Classes	West Berkeley Public Health Center; UC Berkeley Sports Medicine Clinic; Jewish Community Free Clinic (Sonoma County, CA); Goto College of Medical Arts and Sciences (Japan); Shikoku Medical College (Japab); Tianjin University of Traditional Chinese Medicine (China)	English
ACCHS (Academy of Chinese culture and Health Sciences) Oakland	1982 (Taoist Center) 1991 (ACCHS)	1991	MSTCM (Master of Science in Traditional Chinese Medicine)	Certificate: Tuina; Continuing Education		English, Chinese
ACTCM (American College of Traditional Chinese Medicine) San Francisco	1981	1991	MSTCM; DAOM (Doctor of Acupuncture and Oriental Medicine) Specializations: Gynecology; Pain Management	Certificate: Asian Bodywork; Tuina; Shiatsu; Continuing Education	California Pacific Medical Center; Haight Ashbury Free Medical Clinic; Jewish Home for the Aged; UCSF Osher Center for Integrative Medicine; Shanghai University of Traditional Chinese Medicine (China)	English
UEWM (University of East West Medicine) Sunnyvale	1997	2005	MSTCM; Master of Taichi; DAOM (Candidacy with Accreditation Commission) Specializations: Family Medicine; Pain Management	Asian Bodywork; Continuing Education	Beijing University of Chinese Medicine (China); Anhui College of Chinese Medicine (China); Heilongjiang Chinese Medicine University (China)	English, Chinese, Korean

Figure 13.2. TCM Schools in the San Francisco Bay Area. Information in this chart from: California Acupuncture Board Website (http://www.acupuncture.ca.gov/students/schools.shtml), AIMC Website (http://aimc.edu), ACCHS Website: (http://www.acchs.edu), ACTCM Website (http://www.actcm.edu), UEWM Website (http://www.uewm.edu), FBU Website (http://www.fivebranches.edu), and NSUHS Website (http://www.nsuhs.org).

FBU (Five Branches University) Santa Cruz San Jose	1984 (Santa Cruz) 2005 (San Jose)	1996 (Santa Cruz) 2006 (San Jose)	MTCM Optional clinical specializations: Sports Medicine; Tuina Massage; Hepatitis C; Medical Qigong; Yin Tuina) DAOM Specializations: General; Psychotherapy and Psychiatry; Women's Health and Endocrinology; Neuromuscular Medicine and Pain Management; Medical Qigong in Cancer Treatment	Certificate: Asian Bodywork; Qigong Continuing Education	Stanford University; Zhengjiang Medical University (China)	English, Chinese, Korean
NSUHS (Nine Star University of Health Sciences) Sunnyvale	2007	2011	MSOM	Certificate: Massage Practitioner; Massage Therapist; Qigong Instructor; Qigong Master; Acupressure Continuing Education Non-degree Program Public Classes	Henan TCM University (China)	English, Chinese

Figure 13.3. TCM Schools in the San Francisco Bay Area (continued).

Bibliography

PRIMARY SOURCES IN CLASSICAL CHINESE

Baopuzi 抱朴子　Author: Ge Hong 葛洪
Beiji qianjin yaofang 備急千金要方 (Essential Formulae for Emergencies worth a Thousand Pieces of Gold) Author: Sun Simiao 孫思邈
Beiji qianjin yifang 備急千金翼方 (Supplemental Formulae for Emergencies worth a Thousand Pieces of Gold) Author: Sun Simiao 孫思邈
Daode Jing 道德經
Guanzi 管子　Author: Guan Zhong 管仲
Huainanzi 淮南子
Huangdi Neijing Lishu 黃帝內經靈樞 (The Yellow Emperor's Inner Classic: Spiritual Pivot)
Huangdi Neijing Suwen 黃帝內經素問 (The Yellow Emperor's Inner Classic: Basic Questions)
Huangting Neijing Jing 黃庭內景經 (The Inner Radiance Scripture of the Yellow Court)
Liezi 列子　Author: Lie Yukou 列禦寇
Lunheng 論衡 (The Discourse on Balance)　Author: Wang Chong 王充
Lunyu 論語 (The Analects of Confucius)
Zhongheji 中和集 (Collection on the Middle Way)　Author: Li Daochun 李道纯
Zhuangzi 莊子 Author: Zhuang Zhou 莊周
Zhuzi yulei 朱子語類 (Classified Dialogues of Master Zhu)

OTHER WORKS CITED

Ahn, A.C., A.P. Colbert, B.J. Anderson, O.G. Martinsen, R. Hammerschlag, S. Cina, P.M. Wayne, and H.M. Langevin. "Electrical Properties of Acupuncture Points and Meridians: A Systematic Review." *Bioelectromagnetics* 29, no. 4 (2008): 245–56.
Baer, Hans A. *Toward an Integrative Medicine: Merging Alternative Therapies with Biomedicine*. Walnut Creek, CA: AltaMira Press, 2004.
Baer, Hans A., John Hays, Nicole McClendon, Neil McGoldrick, and Raffella Vespucci. "The Holistic Health Movement in the San Francisco Bay Area: Some Preliminary Observations." *Social Science and Medicine* 47, no. 10 (1998): 1495–1501.
Barnes, Linda L. "The Psychologizing of Chinese Healing Practices in the United States." *Culture, Medicine, and Psychiatry* 22 (1998): 413–43.
―――. "The Acupuncture Wars: The Professionalizing of American Acupuncture—a View from Massachusetts." *Medical Anthropology* 22 (2003): 261–301.
―――. "American Acupuncture and Efficacy: Meanings and Their Points of Insertion." *Medical Anthropology Quarterly* 19, no. 3 (2005): 239–66.
Bishop, Shaun. "Palo Alto Acupuncture Pioneer, 82, Dies." *Palo Alto Daily News*, June 30, 2009.
Casanova, Jose. "Religion, the New Millennium, and Globalization." *Sociology of Religion* 62, no. 4 (2001): 415–41.

Cassidy, Claire M. "Chinese Medicine Users in the United States Part I: Utilization, Satisfaction, Medical Plurality." *Journal of Alternative and Complementary Medicine* 4, no. 1 (1998): 17–27.
Center for the Health Professions, University of California, San Francisco. *Acupuncture in California: Study of Scope of Practice*. 2004.
Chen, Hsiang-Shui. *Chinatown No More: Taiwan Immigrants in Contemporary New York*. Ithaca, NY: Cornell University Press, 1992.
Chen, Nancy N. *Breathing Spaces: Qigong, Psychiatry, and Healing in China*. New York Chichester, West Sussex: Columbia University Press, 2003.
Cho, Philip S. *Ritual and the Occult in Chinese Medicine and Religious Healing: The Development of Zhuyou Exorcism*. Dissertation. University of Pennsylvania, 2005.
Clark, Peter A. "The Ethics of Alternative Medicine." *Journal of Public Health Policy* 21, no. 4 (2000): 447–70.
Confucius, and Dim Cheuk Lau. *The Analects*. Harmondsworth; New York: Penguin Books, 1979.
Confucius, and Arthur Waley. *The Analects of Confucius*. New York: Vintage Books, 1989.
Dicker, Laverne Mau. *The Chinese in San Francisco: A Pictorial History*. New York: Dover Publications, 1979.
Emad, Mitra C. "The Debate over Chinese-Language Knowledge among Culture Brokers of Acupuncture in America." *ETC.: A Review of General Semantics* 63, no. 4 (2006): 408–21.
English-Lueck, J. A. *Health in the New Age: A Study in California Holistic Practices*. Albuquerque: University of New Mexico Press, 1990.
Fong, Joe Chung. "Mecca of Chinese American in California: Dai Fow (San Francisco), Yee Fow (Sacramento), and Sam Fow (Stockton)." In *150 Years of the Chinese Presence in California (1848–2001): Honor the Past, Engage the Present, Build the Future*. Sacramento, CA: Sacramento Chinese Culture Foundation; Asian American Studies, University of California, Davis, 2001.
Freedman, Amy L. *Political Participation and Ethnic Minorities: Chinese Overseas in Malaysia, Indonesia, and the United States*. New York: Routledge, 2000.
Fuller, Robert C. *Spiritual, but Not Religious: Understanding Unchurched America*. Oxford; New York: Oxford University Press, 2001.
Gardner, Daniel. *Learning to Be a Sage: Selections from the Conversations of Master Chu, Arranged Topically*. Berkeley: University of California Press, 1990.
Giulianotti, Richard, and Roland Robertson. "Forms of Glocalization: Globalization and the Migration Strategies of Scottish Football Fans in North America." *Sociology of Religion* 41 (2007): 133–52.
Goldstein, Michael S. "The Emerging Socioeconomic and Political Support for Alternative Medicine in the United States." *Annals of the American Academy of Political and Social Science: Global Perspectives on Complemetary and Alternative Medicine*, no. 583 (2002): 44–63.
Gong-Guy, Lillian. *Chinese in San Jose and the Santa Clara Valley*. Chinese Historical and Cultural Project, edited by Lillian Gong-Guy and Gerrye Wong. Charleston, SC: Arcadia Publishing, 2007.
Hammer, Leon. *Dragon Rises and Red Bird Flies: Psychology and Chinese Medicine*. Barrytown, NY: Station Hill Press, 1990.
Hannerz, Ulf. *Cultural Complexity: Studies in the Social Organization of Meaning*. New York and Chichester: Columbia University Press, 1992.
Hare, Martha. "The Emergence of an Urban U.S. Chinese Medicine." *Medical Anthropology Quarterly* 1, no. 1 (1993): 30–49.
Hsu, Elizabeth. "The Reception of Western Medicine into China: Examples from Yunnan." In *Science and Empires*, edited by Patrick Petitjean, Catherine Jami, and Anne Marie Moulin, 89–101. Amsterdam: Kluwer Academic Publishing, 1991.
———. *The Transmission of Chinese Medicine*. Cambridge; NYC; Melbourn: Cambridge Uinversity Press, 1999.

Hu, Fuchen. "The Tri-Level Xing, Qi, Shen Structured Conception of the Body in Daoist Thoughts and Daoist Religion (Daojia He Daojiao Xing Qi Shen Sanchong Jiegou De Rentiguan 道家和道教形，氣，神三重結構的人體觀)." In *Qi Theories and Conception of the Body in Ancient Chinese Thoughts (Zhongguo Gudai Sixiang Zhong De Qilun Ju Shentiguan 中國古代思想中的氣論及身體觀)*, edited by Ru-Bin Yang, 171–76. Taipei: Juliu Publishing, 1993.

Hui, K.K., E.E. Nixon, M.G. Vangel, J. Liu, O. Marina, V. Napadow, S.M. Hodge, B.R. Rosen, N. Makris, and D.N. Kennedy. "Characterization of The 'Deqi' Response in Acupuncture." *BMC Complementary Alternative Medicine* 7, no. 33 (2007).

Ishida, Hideme. "Looking at the Characteristics of Ancient Chinese View of the Body through the Knowledge of the Development Process of the Body (You Shenti Shengcheng Guocheng De Renshi Laikan Zhongguo Gudai Shentiguan De Tezhi 由身體生成過程的認識來看中國古代身體觀的特質)." In *Qi Theories and Conception of the Body in Ancient Chinese Thoughts (Zhongguo Gudai Sixiang Zhong De Qilun Ju Shentiguan 中國古代思想中的氣論及身體觀)*, edited by Ru-Bin Yang, 177–92. Taipei: Juliu Publishing, 1993.

Kaptchuk, Ted. J. *The Web That Has No Weaver: Understanding Chinese Medicine*. New York: McGraw-Hill, 2000.

Kohn, Livia. *Daoism and Chinese Culture*. Cambridge, MA: Three Pine Press, 2001.

Kong, J., R. Gollub, G. Polich, V. Napadow, K. Hui, M. Vangel, B. Rosen, and Ted. J. Kaptchuk. "Acupuncture De Qi, from Qualitative History to Quantitative Measurement." *Journal of Alternative and Complementary Medicine* 13, no. 10 (2007): 1059–70.

Korom, Frank. "Memory, Innovation and Emergent Ethnicities." *Diaspora* 3, no. 2 (1994): 135–55.

Kwong, Peter. *The New Chinatown*. New York: Hill and Wang, 1996.

Laozi, D. T. Suzuki, and Paul Carus. *Treatise on Response and Retribution*. La Salle, IL: Open Court Publishing, 1973.

Lau, Kimberly J. *New Age Capitalism: Making Money East of Eden*. Philadelphia: University of Pennsylvania Press, 2000.

Lee, Miriam. *Insights of a Senior Acupuncturist*. Boulder: Blue Poppy Press, 1992.

Legge, James. *Confucian Analects*. Whitefish, MT: Kessinger Publishing, 2004.

Li, Yongming, "The War between Dragon and Snake: The Birth of First Legalization of Traditional Chinese Medicine in the United States (Longshe Dazhan: Meiguo Diyige Zhongyifa De Dansheng 龍蛇大戰：美國第一個中醫法的誕生)." *World Journal Weekend Special*, March 9, 2008.

Liu, Lihong. *Thoughts on Chinese Medicine (Sikao Zhongyi 思考中醫)*. Taipei: Jimu Wenhua Publishing, 2004.

Lu, Gwei-djen, and Joseph Needham. *Celestial Lancets: A History and Rationale of Acupuncture and Moxa*. Cambridge: Cambridge University Press, 1980.

MacPherson, H., and A. Asghar. "Acupuncture Needle Sensations Associated with De Qi: A Classification Based on Experts' Ratings." *Journal of Alternative and Complementary Medicine* 12, no. 7 (2006): 633–37.

Mao, J. J., J.T. Farrar, K. Armstrong, A. Donahue, J. Ngo, and M.A. Bowman. "De Qi: Chinese Acupuncture Patients' Experiences and Beliefs Regarding Acupuncture Needling Sensation—an Exploratory Survey." *Acupuncture Medicine* 25, no. 4 (2007): 158–65.

Nahin, Richard L., Patricia M. Barnes, Barbara J. Strussman, and Barbara Bloom. *Cost of Complementary and Alternative Medicine (Cam) and Frequency of Visits to Cam Practitioners: United States, 2007*. U.S. Department of Health and Human Services, Centers for Disease Control and Prevention, and National Center for Health Statistics, 2009.

O'Connor, Bonnie B. *Healing Traditions: Alternative Medicine and the Health Professions*. Philadelphia: University of Pennsylvania Press, 1995.

Paulus, Wolfgang, and Mingmin Zhang. "Influence of Acupuncture on the Pregnancy Rate in Patients Who Undergo Assisted Reproduction Therapy." *Fertility and Sterility* 77, no. 4 (2002): 721–24.

Prothero, Stephen. *American Jesus: How the Son of God Became a National Icon*. New York: Farrar, Straus and Giroux, 2003.

Reston, James. "Now, Let Me Tell You About My Appendectomy in Peking." *The New York Times* (July 26, 1971), 1 and 6.

Robertson, Roland. "Glocalization: Time-Space and Homogeneity-Heterogeneity." In *Global Modernities*, edited by Mike Featherstone, Scott Lash, and Roland Robertson, 25–44. London: Sage Publications, 1995.

Roof, Wade Clark. *Spiritual Marketplace: Baby Boomers and the Remaking of American Religion*. Princeton: Princeton University Press, 1999.

Roudometof, Victor. "Transnationalism, Cosmopolitanism and Glocalization." *Current Sociology* 53, no. 1 (2005): 113–35.

Sangren, Paul Steven. *History and Magical Power in a Chinese Community*. Stanford: Stanford University Press, 1987.

Scheid, Volker. *Chinese Medicine in Contemporary China: Plurality and Synthesis*. Durham; London: Duke University Press, 2002.

———. "Remodeling the Arsenal of Chinese Medicine: Shared Pasts, Alternative Futures." *Annals of the American Academy of Political and Social Science: Global Perspectives on Complementary and Alternative Medicine* 583 (2002): 136–59.

Schwartz, Robert. "Acupuncture and Expertise: A Challenge to Physician Control." *The Hastings Center Report* 11, no. 2 (1981): 5–7.

Sharf, Robert H. *Coming to Terms with Chinese Buddhism: A Reading of the Treasure Store Treatise*. Honolulu: University of Hawai'i Press, 2002.

Shils, Edward. *Center and Periphery: Essays in Macro Society*. Chicago: University of Chicago Press, 1975.

Sivin, Nathan. *Traditional Medicine in Contemporary China*. Ann Arbor: Center for Chinese Studies, University of Michigan, 1987.

Spitzer, Nicholas R. "Monde Créole: The Cultural World of French Louisiana Creoles and the Creolization of World Cultures." *Journal of American Folklore* 116, no. 459 (2003): 57–72.

Stark, Rodney, and Roger Finke. *Acts of Faith: Explaining the Human Side of Religion*. Berkeley: University of California Press, 2000.

Tambiah, Stanley J. "Transnational Movements, Diaspora, and Multiple Modernities." *Daedalus* 129, no. 1 (2000): 163–94.

Tölölyan, Khachig. "Rethinking Diaspora(s): Stateless Power in the Transnational Moment." *Diaspora* 5, no. 1 (1996): 3–36.

Tomlinson, John *Globalization and Culture*. Cambridge: Polity, 1999.

Turner, Victor. *The Ritual Process: Structure and Anti-Structure Symbol, Myth, and Ritual*, edited by Victor Turner. Ithaca: Cornell University Press, 1969.

Unschuld, Paul U. *Medicine in China: A History of Ideas*. Berkeley; Los Angeles; London: University of California Press, 1985.

Wey, Nancy. "A History of Chinese Americans in California." *Five Views: An Ethnic Historic Site Survey for California* (1988). http://www.nps.gov/history/history/online_books/5views/5views3.htm (accessed November 14, 2009).

Wuthnow, Robert. *After Heaven: Spirituality in America since the 1950s*. Berkeley: University of California Press, 1998.

Yao, Xingzhong. *An Introduction to Confucianism*. New York: Cambridge University Press, 2000.

Zhan, Mei. "Does It Take a Miracle? Negotiating Knowledges, Identities, and Communities of Traditional Chinese Medicine." *Cultural Anthropology* 16, no. 4 (2001): 453–80.

Index

acupuncture, 5, 12n6, 26, 30–31, 144, 204; American, 30; Anesthesia, 30; community, 51–55; ear; auricular, 52–53; Five Elements, 61; French, 30; infertility treatment, 118–120; Japanese, 30, 105–106, 111; Korean, 30, 166, 169; Legalization, 43n9, 43n10; pain management; Vietnamese, 30. *See also* community clinic; Working Class Acupuncture

Acupuncture Association of America (AAA), 33

acupuncture licensing, 30, 43n10, 46; California requirements, 26, 46, 55, 64–65, 71; California scope of practice, 26, 75; Nevada legislation, 30–31

acupuncture schools: Chinese program, 47–48, 48–50, 66; clinical training, 46, 50–51; curricula, 64–65; curricular models, 66–67; English program, 47–48, 50, 66; internship in China, 73; internship in school clinic, 73; school clinic, 50–51, 52–53; schools in Bay Area, 64, 66–67, 227, 228; teaching format, 48–50; teaching styles, 48–50

acupuncturists in California, 5; demographics, 21–22; religious identities and affiliations, 22; spiritual practices, 22

Adam (pseudonym), 69, 103, 105–106, 107, 107–108, 109, 109, 110

AIDS epidemic, 32, 36, 37, 54, 165

Aikido 合気道, 93

Albert (pseudonym), 84–87, 88

Alison (pseudonym), 55, 60–61, 138–141, 149, 209

American Board of Oriental Reproductive Medicine (ABROM), 118

apprenticeship, 71–73

Ashley, 152, 163–170, 196–197, 208

Bodhisattva Guanyin, 127, 128, 131n9

California State Acupuncture Board, 46, 64, 71

cause of disease, 25, 109, 126–127, 136, 151–154, 154–155, 169, 175–176, 181, 218

Charles (pseudonym), 120–124, 129, 130

Chinatowns, 19–20, 29

Chinese American, 18

Chinese diaspora, 18. *See also* diaspora

Chinese Exclusion Act, 17, 29

chiropractic, 121, 123, 124

Chris (pseudonym), 93–96, 99, 100

clairvoyance, 86, 122

classical formulae (jingfang 經方), 143, 144

clinic ambience, 148–150

clinical practices, 24–25

clinical procedure, 168, 199

cold (han 寒), 126, 127

community clinic, 51–55, 68, 101, 140, 148

complementary and alternative medicine (CAM), 5

Confucian value, 34–35

Confucius, 175

correspondence theory, 153–154, 177, 178, 184–185

Creolization, 212–213

Crystal (pseudonym), 35–37, 41, 43n18, 193, 207

cultivation methods, 22–23, 177, 218. *See also* taichi *and* taichi quan

Cultural Revolution, 18

Dao, 178
deep ecology, 160n3
deqi 得氣, 181, 181–182, 186, 188n27, 206
diagnosis, 50–51; dowsing rod, 120; psychic, 120, 121–122, 126–127; pulse, 50, 78, 80, 127; remote, 125; TCM, 50–51, 94, 98, 181; tongue, 80
diaspora, 27n8
disease. *See* cause of disease
Doctor of Oriental Medicine (OMD), 9, 79
Dr. Hsieh (pseudonym), 155–156, 160
Dr. Yuan (pseudonym), 113–115, 179, 181, 181–182
Dr. Zhang (pseudonym), 124–129, 130, 193

earth (di 地), 177
energetic IQ, 120
energy healing, 24, 166, 204
energy sensation. *See* qi, sensations
environmental issues, 153–154
Estelle (pseudonym), 150, 165
ethnic diversity, 16
exorcism, 109, 128
experiential dimension, 206
Experts' Clinic, 56–57

Falungong 法輪功, 210
fengshui 風水, 85–86, 88n11, 148, 149, 158
Five Elements, 12n17, 60, 147, 174, 177, 184, 192, 199
food therapy, 124, 127, 156, 158
free clinic, 54, 112, 139, 140, 165

ganying 感應 (empathetic resonance), 181, 185
Ge Hong 葛洪, 176–177
George (pseudonym), 61–62, 142–145, 145, 152–154, 192
ghost (gui 鬼), 109, 128–129
ghost points, 109
globalization, 212
Guanyin. *See* Bodhisattva Guanyin
Guan Zhong 管仲, 175
Gu Daifu (pseudonym), 78–81, 88

healing, 189
health, 189, 189, 190; definitions, 189, 190, 200
heaven (tian 天), 177
herbalist, 78–81
herbology, 78, 144
hereditary physicians, 46
holism, 12n19, 91, 129, 134, 146, 160, 184
holistic medicine, 5, 25, 89, 91–92, 107, 110, 117, 138, 154, 189, 207
homeopathy, 97
Huangdi Neijing 黃帝內經, 58, 60, 144, 175
Huangting Jing 黃庭經, 191

identity formation, 67–70
ideological conversion, 206
integrative medicine, 59, 60, 66, 73, 92, 94, 96–97, 120

Jason (pseudonym), 32, 38–40, 42, 43n19, 56–57, 179–180, 181, 208
jing 精 (essence), 126, 153, 177, 178, 186, 195
jing 敬 (reverence), 178
jing qi shen 精氣神, 135, 172, 177, 178, 195
Jingshen 精神, 39, 171, 172–173, 174, 178, 194
Jingye 津液 (body fluid), 80
Jinkui Yaolue 金匱要略, 58, 143
Joy (pseudonym), 103–105, 107, 108, 109, 109, 115, 208

Kang Youwei 康有為, 171
Kelly (pseudonym), 60, 96–99, 101
knowledge transmission, 45–46, 47–48, 55–57; challenges in TCM schools, 55–57; Chinese medical classics, 57–62
Krause, Art, 33

Lee, Miriam, 32–33, 34, 35, 36, 37, 38, 40–41, 42, 43n11, 43n12, 43n14
Li 理 (principle), 178
Lie Yukou 列禦寇, 176
lifestyle changes, 154–155, 158–160
Linda (pseudonym), 76–78, 87

Ling 靈, 172
literati physicians, 46
localization, 212
Lok Yee Kung 陸易公, 31

manual therapy, 81–82, 155
martial arts. *See* Aikido; Shintaido
master-disciple relationship, 72–73
Master Lin (pseudonym), 157–160
Master Tung's Points, 43n12, 166, 169
medical acupuncture, 95
medical qigong, 125, 152, 169
Meilun (pseudonym), 59–60, 173, 182
Meridians, 80, 107, 108, 120, 126, 127, 144, 169, 174, 182, 184, 186, 190, 192, 193, 194, 199
Ming (pseudonym), 70
Mou Zongsan 牟宗三, 33
Mt. Emei, 166, 170n1
mysterious (xuan 玄), 171, 179

National Certification Commission for Acupuncture and Oriental Medicine (NCCAOM), 71
National Institute of Health (NIH), 204
Nixon, Richard, 30
non-profit clinic. *See* free clinic

Oriental medicine, 9, 46

pain management, 93
patent medicine, 81
Paul (pseudonym), 68–69
physical body: shen 身, 177; ti 體, 177–178
Pigu 辟穀 (abstinence from grains), 197
practical formulae (shifang 實方), 143
practitioner of Chinese medicine (Zhongyi 中醫; zhongyishi 中醫師), 7
prayer, 107
private apprenticeship. *See* apprenticeship

qi, 60, 147, 174–176, 205, 211; blockage, 169, 194; cosmic, 196, 200, 209; cultivation, 83, 116, 128, 195, 196–197; deficiency, 193; definitions, 60, 147, 171, 174, 175, 209; diseased (bingqi 病氣), 151, 152; evil, 128, 194; han 寒氣 (cold qi), 126, 128; infusion, 83–84, 166, 169; leakage, 194, 195; managing (yingqi 營氣), 126; model: battery, 194, 194; model: irrigation, 190; model: management, 190–191, 199; plum pit, 183; pollution, 151–154; protective (weiqi 衛氣), 126, 128; refinement, 177, 186, 195, 200; sensations, 63, 180, 181–183, 186; stagnation, 181; yangqi 陽氣, 153, 195
qigong, 23, 83, 86–87, 127, 138, 156, 164, 166, 186, 194, 196–197, 210
quiet sitting,. *See also* sitting meditation 23, 178

Rafael (pseudonym), 63, 133–138, 145, 150–151, 209
religion, 22, 25, 40, 136–137, 140, 180, 211
religiosity (zongjiao 宗教), 83, 171–172, 173, 180
Reston, James, 30
ritual: definition, 24, 28n17; healing, 84, 166, 169; practices, 86

Sally (pseudonym), 152
San Francisco/Bay Area, 15–20
scientific, 159, 166, 174, 179–180, 181
senior practitioners. *See* Experts' Clinic
Shanghan Lun 傷寒論, 58, 142, 144
shen 神 (miraculous), 179, 181
shen 神 (spirit), 135, 175, 176, 177, 178, 178, 181, 186, 194, 195
shen 身. *See* physical body
shenming 神明 (deities), 209
Shintaido, 111
sitting meditation, 23, 178, 218
Sophia (pseudonym), 33–35, 41, 43n15, 172, 174, 207
spirit possession, 128–129
spiritual: cultivation, 25, 150, 161n6, 200; definition, 25, 133, 138, 171–174, 186, 207, 211; dimension, 89, 107–110, 130, 134, 136, 206, 207, 209, 214–211; resources, 25, 129, 208, 209, 211, 214

spirituality, 25, 106–107, 123, 136, 137, 138, 174, 207, 210
Steinberg, Arthur, 31
Su Daifu (pseudonym), 72–73, 81–84, 88
Sun Simiao 孫思邈, 135, 146n3
superstition, 84, 171, 173, 175

taichi, 23, 28n16, 104, 137, 161n6, 164, 222
taichi quan (taiji quan 太極拳), 164
Tara (pseudonym), 117–120, 129, 130
tea master, 157
Thomas (pseudonym), 89–93, 99–100
ti 體. *See* physical body
Traditional Chinese Medicine (TCM): as alternative medicine, 25; in American mainstream, 8; in Chinese American community, 8; in Chinese civilization, 7–47; classical, 61–62, 142, 145; definition, 1, 6, 7, 8; energetic aspect, 61, 63; integrative TCM, 96–99, 114; modern, 142; in PRC (PRC-TCM), 6, 61, 76, 113–114; veterinarian, 91
traditional Chinese medical school. *See* acupuncture school
transformation, 24; emotional, 24; energetic, 148–150; psychological, 24; spiritual, 150, 186; qi, 177, 178, 186
transnationalism, 17
tuina 推拿 (massage therapy). *See* manual therapy

Vera (pseudonym), 52–53, 110–112, 115
vitalism, 9

Wang Chong 王充, 178
Wei (pseudonym), 70
Working Class Acupuncture, 54. *See also* acupuncture, community; community clinic

Xin 心 (heart-mind), 176
xing 形 (physical form), 176, 177, 177–178, 195

yang organ (fu 腑), 184, 192
Yang Wei-chieh 楊維傑, 43n12
Yiguandao 一貫道, 124, 128, 129, 130n7
Yijing 易經, 135
yin organ (zang 臟), 184, 192
yinyang 陰陽, 137, 138, 147, 174, 177, 185, 186, 192, 193, 200

zhenggu 整骨 (skeletomuscular adjustments). *See* manual therapy
Zhuang Zhou 莊周, 175
Zhu Xi 朱熹, 178

About the Author

Emily S. Wu has a PhD in Cultural and Historical Studies of Religions from the Graduate Theological Union in Berkeley, with specializations in Chinese folk religions and Daoism. Her current research primarily focuses on Chinese and Chinese American religious practices and beliefs that intersect with medicine, healing, and understandings of the human body. As a college instructor in the San Francisco Bay Area, she also teaches undergraduate and graduate courses in Asian religions and cultures.